Posture Alignment

The Missing Link in Health and Fitness

Paul D'Arezzo, M.D.

Illustrations by Nathanael Letteer

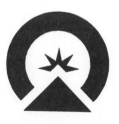

Marcellina Mountain Press
Colorado Springs, Colorado

For Malia and Matthew

About the Author:

Paul D'Arezzo, M.D. is a board-certified emergency physician having practiced in Virginia, Florida, Hawaii, and Colorado. Over many years after seeing countless patients with muscle and joint complaints, he became interested in the effects of body alignment on muscle and joint health and function. Combining his extensive medical background with yoga and other disciplines, he presents a clear case for the need for correcting and maintaining our posture. He is currently a postural alignment specialist residing in Colorado Springs, Colorado.

Acknowledgements:

- To my family and friends, particularly Carol, Vivian, and Rebecca, for all their support and encouragement.

- To Nathanael Letteer for his wonderful illustrations.

- To all the patients I have treated and the health professionals I have had the privilege to work with — thank you.

- To my yoga teachers — Namaste.

Disclaimer: This book is not a substitute for professional healthcare and makes no claims and takes no responsibility for the results any given individual may obtain by following the prescribed advice or exercise programs. As always if you have any underlying medical conditions or are older, it is always prudent to seek the advice of your doctor or healthcare provider before initiating any exercise program. Also, as in all situations, listen to your own body and use your own best judgment.

Published by Marcellina Mountain Press
        P.O. Box 6781
        Colorado Springs, CO 80934

Website: www.posturealignment.com

Illustrations by Nathanael Letteer

Design and layout by Dina Snow, Azteca Design

ISBN 0-9729079-0-4

Library of Congress Control Number: 2003103498

Printed by Hignell Book Printing in Canada

Table of Contents

Introduction

Just look around. We've become a nation of walking wounded. We slouch, we waddle, we sag. We collapse into our chairs and hunch over our desks and computers. More and more of us are looking crooked, rounded, and just generally out-of-line at earlier and earlier ages. And it hurts us and is killing us.

Because posture is more than just something that looks pretty. While most people know that posture involves appearance, fewer are aware that our posture or body alignment is also intimately connected to function—with what we can or can not physically do—and particularly as we grow older with muscle and joint pain and disability.

You may have justifiably picked up this book, however, because you don't like the way you look. You may look slouched, collapsed, or hunched over. You might not look as healthy as you'd like. You might be beginning to look like your parents or grandparents long before you think you should.

Like it or not, we are both judged and judge others by their posture. Those with more erect posture are perceived as happier, more confident, and more in control. Older people with good posture are perceived as younger.

No matter what your age, Posture Alignment will improve your appearance. You will look younger. People will notice a difference in the way you look and move.

Or you may find yourself unable to do things you used to do. With age there is gradual erosion in our physical ability. We tend to give up sports and activities we once loved. If we aren't careful, it becomes harder to do simple things—walking up stairs can become a burden, getting down on the floor can become an impossibility. But all of this loss of function is not inevitable. There are things we can do to forestall it.

As you will see, with deterioration in our body's alignment, there is also a disinclination to be active. It is no longer fun or comfortable. Posture Alignment can reverse these things. When we restore our lost alignment, we feel a surge in health.

Or you may have been through a long progression of doctors, healthcare providers, or exercise programs. No one seems to know what's going on; nothing seems to help. As a physician, over a number of years I've come to believe that a great deal of our muscle and joint injuries and problems—including the current epidemic of carpal tunnel, rotator cuff disorders, back pain, knee and ankle disorders—have its root causes in our loss of alignment. When our joints and muscles are out of alignment it causes pain. Posture Alignment may be the thing you need to help.

Simple exercise can't solve all our problems. Unless we do something to correct our alignment first, most exercise and activity will only tend to reinforce or perpetuate any dysfunction. That's why Posture Alignment is the missing link in health and fitness.

The first part of this book presents the principles of body alignment. I've purposely avoided the game of muscle-naming and scientific jargon. The principles underlying the function of our muscles, joints, and alignment are simple and can be understood by a child.

Following this is a self-assessment where you get to take a closer look at your own posture and alignment. Then exercises are prescribed in menus to help correct specific alterations in your posture. If your back or shoulders are rounded forward, there are exercises to correct that. If your knees, ankles, or feet hurt, there are exercises that can help.

Page through the book and you will notice some of the exercises are different than ones you may be used to. The goal of the exercises isn't to run you through your paces, but rather to slowly, gradually correct areas of stiffness and weakness and bring your body back into alignment.

The final chapter presents some new alternative ways of thinking about health and fitness to help you preserve function into the next decades as you grow older.

But there are no magic cures. All the technology and modern medicine— all the king's horses and all the king's men—can't put you back together and keep you there. You will have to put yourself back together. This will take a little effort. But it is worth it.

While I don't claim these exercises will absolutely, positively correct any and all posture abnormalities (for many people, they will), I do claim when done properly they will move anyone strongly in the direction of correct postural alignment. They are powerful tools. You *will* look and feel better. You *will* move better.

Finally remember this isn't an all or nothing proposition. Anything you can do to improve and maintain your body's alignment is worthwhile. A small correction in your alignment can make you look and feel years younger. A little correction in your alignment may be enough to get rid of a pain which has been plaguing you for years. Improving your posture may allow you to keep doing activities you might otherwise have given up.

So let's get started.

CHAPTER 1

The Problem

We are not getting old—we are developing powerful muscles which allow us to sit for long periods of time without getting tired.

– Quote on a coffee mug

Funny, huh? But if we aren't careful, as we grow older, our reality may go something like this.

You will get older and stiffer. You will stop participating in sports and other physical activities you used to enjoy. You'll say "I just don't have time anymore" or make up some other reason, but the real reason will be they are no longer fun or easy to do. Your body can no longer comfortably do them.

With more time, simple things that you used to do like bending over to pick something up off the floor or walking up several flights of stairs will become more of an effort. You'll avoid those things if you can. It will become harder to get up when you sit down. You won't like going up or down stairs. There is going to be more creaking in your joints.

You may even hear yourself saying things like, "I don't like stairs anymore," "I can't sit in that type chair," or "Drop me off at the entrance, I don't like walking."

You'll probably develop pain in your neck, shoulders, back, or knees. You will see doctors. There will be X rays. You'll be prescribed pain medicines. Maybe there will be surgery or even joint replacement surgery.

In the midst of all this you may decide you need to exercise again. You will take out your old jogging shoes, try to take up your old sport again, or do the exercises from some magazine article you read. It will help a little but the progression will continue. Maybe you just didn't do it enough.

Throw in a few visits to a chiropractor for some relief. The injuries or pain may go away for awhile but they will come back, or come back in different places. Your physical well-being will continue to deteriorate. You will physically be able to do less and less.

You may blame all this on normal aging, a fact of life, bad genes, or simply bad luck. But without knowing it, you will be throwing in the towel long before your time.

The loss of function will continue. It will worry you. You've been active your whole life. You've never been a couch potato. And you have a lot of years left to live. If this is happening now, what is it going to be like ten or twenty or more years from now? At first this musculoskeletal loss of function may be just an inconvenience, a nuisance that limits you. But eventually it may reach a point where you are in constant pain and it demands your full attention. It may severely limit what you can or can not do. And maybe you are only in your forties or fifties or even younger.

Like the ghost of Christmas future in *A Christmas Carol* I present a bleak picture.

The Downward Spiral

This almost invariable downhill slide in our physical function, I term the downward spiral. It is the gradual, insidious loss of functional body movement often accompanied by joint and muscle aches, pains, and disability.

We stop doing things because they are no longer easy to do or because it hurts or becomes uncomfortable to do them. Like an environmental poison, this loss of function sneaks up on us. And while any given point in this downward spiral may seem like an isolated event, they are all related. Each leads to and sets the stage for the next.

> Loss of physical function sneaks up
> on us like an environmental poison.

Surely, it shouldn't matter that we stopped playing softball or tennis or hiking. Or that we've become reluctant to bend down to pick something up off the floor? Or have trouble getting our shoes on? Or that our back or knees hurt? Is there any connection between all these things? You bet there is. Each of these singular events should ring loud warning bells in our minds.

Often only when something big happens—an injury or a disability—do we become aware that something may have been happening beneath the surface for a long time.

Think back over the past five or ten years of your life. Like paging through a photo album, you might be able to pinpoint the date of an injury, or the date you gave up or stopped doing certain activities or could no longer comfortably do them.

"Here I stopped playing basketball," "Here it became hard to get up out of a chair," "Here I had my knee surgery and stopped doing this," "Here I made a conscious decision not to do that anymore because it was too hard or too uncomfortable."

Here is a picture of the downward spiral in case you don't get the idea:

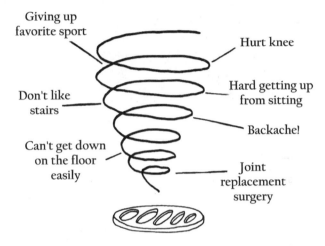

It's Cumulative

Any physical activity or function that you give up now may very well remain lost for the rest of your life. And more will be lost on top of that. If your knee hurts and you give up running, there is a very real possibility that you won't take it up again.

And it goes for simple things as well. If you stop or only rarely get down on the floor, getting down on the floor will become something you avoid or don't do. You will lose the ability to comfortably do that. If you have trouble going up more than three flights of stairs, that will become two flights of stairs. Soon another layer of limitation will be added on top of that. Now you will have trouble getting up from sitting down *and* have trouble lifting your feet to put on your shoes. Again, are they related? Of course they are; they use similar muscles. It will take some time for the weakness to progress. Then you decide not to walk up stairs at all. And it goes on. Like the last stands of trees in a forest being cut down.

> Whatever musculoskeletal function
> you lose or give up now, that will remain
> lost and you will lose more on top of that.

This should give one pause. Whenever I see or hear of people becoming more limited in their movement, I think, "Maybe you don't want to throw that away so soon. Maybe you'll need that or want that in the future."

Don't begin heaving things out of your life raft before you know how long you'll be at sea.

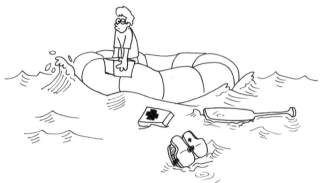

You might need that, you know.

In the midst of all this you may get a wake-up call.

The Wake-Up Call

We've all had them. If you haven't, you probably will. The wake-up call is an event when you come face to face with this deterioration in your physical ability. Maybe a wake-up call made you pick up this book.

One of mine occurred one day crossing a street. You know the feeling: you see the car coming from way off and you think you can make it across before it gets to you. The light was green but I felt I had plenty of time to make it. I took off running (I don't run) and running was suddenly not what I remembered it to be. My legs felt like lead. My body felt heavy and uncoordinated. There was a disconnected feeling of my mind remembering what my body used to be able to do and expecting it and my body suddenly not up to the challenge.

The thought flashed through my mind, "I'm not going to make it!"
The driver didn't slow down; pedestrians are fair game where I live.

I did make it. And I wasn't so much mad at the driver, or even that I had gotten older but just more shocked with how much my physical abilities had deteriorated without me being aware of it.

Often a wake-up call is an injury, or joint or muscle pain that lays you up for longer than you'd expect, or becomes a persistent part of your life. Or the back pain that laid you, "the man" or woman, out for two weeks. Or you find yourself requiring orthopedic surgery of some sort.

Maybe a wake-up call happens when you try to participate in a sport you haven't played in a long time. Suddenly the bat is heavier; second base is a lot farther away than it used to be. Or you go skiing and it turns into a frightful experience. Or you work in the yard and the old back isn't what it used to be.

Or it doesn't have to be something so dramatic. It may just be not being able to reach up to the top shelf as easily anymore. Or more pain getting in and out of a car. Or being unable to get down on the floor to play with your kid. Or feeling or moving or making noises like your parents did.

Or you don't like how you look. Maybe you suddenly see yourself in a mirror and you don't like what you see. You look older than you should. You look shorter. You look sagging and collapsed. Your posture makes you look like your parents or grandparents long before you think you should. You don't look as healthy or as vibrant as you'd like. And you'd like to do something about it.

The wake-up call is something that gets your attention. We all get them but we don't always listen.

At this point, you make a decision. Depending on your background, your beliefs about fitness or health, you chuck up the discomfort, disability, or change in appearance to just getting old or simply being out of shape. You tell yourself you could get back into shape if you wanted to or had the time.

What Used To Work Doesn't Work Anymore

Maybe at this point, something in you wakes up with the wake-up call. You try to do something. You take up jogging again. For two weeks you wake up an hour early and run around a local track. But it just doesn't feel or good. It doesn't feel like it used to. Your knee hurts. Your back hurts. Your feet hurt. You just don't seem to be able to get back into shape like you used to.

Maybe it is just a matter of doing it more. You do it more. It never used to hurt this bad. But despite your best efforts, it keeps hurting and you just don't like it. Sooner or later you drop it.

> ### What used to work doesn't work anymore.

You are now in a precarious position. What used to work to "get you back into shape" doesn't work. What now? Maybe you should take up yoga or stretching—something more benign. You may do that for a while and get some results, but the slide continues. Even if you do get some results, you reach a certain point where you can go no further.

> ### You want to do something to make
> ### it better but you don't know what to do.

Normal Aging

At this point, many people would suggest that all or most of what I describe above is simply normal aging. Hey, it happens. We see it all around us. It's to be expected. It is a fact of life.

I agree. I agree that it happens and I agree that most people expect it. But the premise of this book is that it doesn't have to happen or at least not to the degree that it is happening, or at such early ages.

> Much of our loss of function is NOT
> normal aging. It may be commonplace
> but it doesn't have to be that way.

What are the parameters of normal aging anyway? I dunno. Seriously, I don't know and I'm not sure anyone else does either. Scientific studies can delineate a broad range of what is observed happening to people as they age. But it is often difficult to decide what is incontrovertible biological principle and what has to do with what we do or do not do.

Tissues do lose water and get stiffer as we get older. But a huge part of what falls under the category of normal aging is simply the combined results, as I will show you, of loss of muscle strength, flexibility, and alignment. In most cases, one doesn't need to evoke the latest National Institutes of Health studies on aging to find the cause of our collapsing physical selves. We don't move enough, we have become weak and stiff, and our bodies have gotten out of alignment.

Another scary thing about the aging argument is: What if we are accepting or allowing ourselves to deteriorate before we are really required to? What if we could do some things to prevent or at least dramatically postpone this? Would that be worthwhile?

> If you could do anything to postpone, put off,
> or not have to go through with the downward
> spiral, would that be worthwhile?

What Makes Us Look Old Anyway?

What makes a person look old anyway? Sure it shows in our face and hair and skin (but plastic surgeons are doing all they can about that). To a large degree what makes a person look old is how they move. Or to be more accurate, how they don't move.

In a word, the old (whatever age you pick for that) are stiff and inflexible. When they sit down, it is hard to get up. It is hard to reach under the table to pick something up. They move in limited set ranges of movement. The physical aging process can be seen in great part as a gradual limitation in our movement potential.

> Looking old (whatever age you pick) is in great part related to how we are able to move, or not move.

Part of what we fear most about getting old is this restriction in movement. Studies show that what people fear most is not dying but being disabled. We can't or won't be able to do everything we want to. Having our biological basis as hunting, gathering, moving animals, lack of mobility strikes at our evolutionary core. Like any animal, we have an intuitive sense that our life depends on movement. We know that to stop moving is to die. The downward spiral strikes at our evolutionary core. Loss of function is a gradual form of disability.

> To stop moving is to die.

What Causes The Downward Spiral?

Simply put, as we grow older not only do we move less but also we move with less variety. Most often this is due to a job and lifestyle that don't require much real movement or only the same repetitive movements. We sit in our cars, we drive to work, we sit at work or walk a little, and then we drive home. The bottom line is we aren't moving enough and with enough variety to keep ourselves functional. We don't bend, stoop, reach, or stretch very much or very far. We don't lift or carry much weight very often.

> We don't move enough and with enough variety to keep ourselves functional.

And if you think about it, is it really surprising that we have trouble doing something we only do once a week or once a month or twice a year? Is it really surprising that muscles we don't use get weak and then we are surprised at walking and moving like old people? I mean, if you never or rarely get down on the floor and crawl is it surprising that that becomes hard to do. Where is the mystery here?

If we don't move with enough variety, some muscles become stiff.

Think of your normal range of stretching and reaching for things as a box or a three-dimensional volume of space around you.

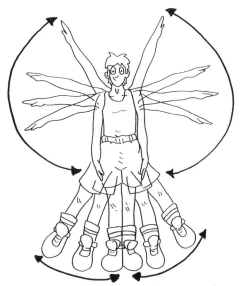

Area in which we can comfortably
reach and stretch

As we grow older, this box becomes smaller. We reach or stretch into its peripheries less often. We don't become stiff for no reason. We become stiff because we stop stretching outside our normal ranges. The mantra of all life is "use it or lose it." Muscles that we don't use become stiff; they lose their ability to stretch and extend to the farthest reaches of their kingdoms. Our normal range of motion, and our world, becomes smaller.

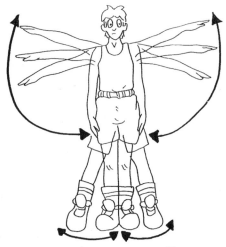

Area becoming smaller

> ## Some of our muscles have become stiff.

The second thing that occurs is that certain muscles that we don't commonly use but still need get weak. We aren't required to carry significant weight very often. We sit a lot. Some muscles are used a lot, some hardly at all. Any muscle that isn't routinely used becomes weak. Stronger, more-used muscles dominate weaker, under-used muscles.

We often underestimate this diminution in our muscular strength. Unfortunately, most of us are much weaker than we think in a number of key muscle groups.

> ## Some of our muscles have become weak.

Most people may be aware, at least on some level, of the above two things occurring: some muscles becoming stiff and losing their range of motion and other muscles becoming weak. But we are often not aware of the consequence of these two things. They set the stage for a bad thing to begin to happen. Our postural alignment begins to collapse.

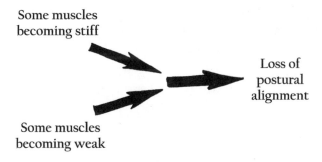

> ## Some muscles becoming stiff and some muscles becoming weak lead to alterations in our postural alignment.

Why Is Postural Alignment Important?

All machinery is designed to work with a specific alignment. If the design parameters of the machine are violated or the parts become mal-aligned, things don't work the way they should. Parts grind and grate and there is accelerated wear and tear.

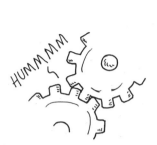

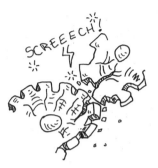

Aligned parts work smoothly   Mal-aligned parts <u>don't</u>

It is the same with our human bodies. Our spines and major weight-bearing joints are designed to operate with a specific alignment. If our postural alignment begins to collapse, things don't work the way they should. For us, as humans, this translates into a disinclination to be physically active and can result in pain and disability.

In this book, I use the words 'posture' or 'postural alignment' to describe the anatomically correct alignment of our spines and joints—the way our joints and muscles are designed to line-up for us to function optimally. Other equally valid phrases might be 'structural alignment' or 'functional alignment'. I use the term *Posture Alignment* to describe the method of correcting any aberrations in our posture.

Here is an overview of some of the key points in this correct postural alignment that allows optimal functioning of our bodies.

Our bodies are designed to be aligned vertically with gravity, that is, not leaning or bending too far forward or backward.

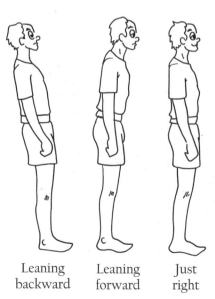

Leaning   Leaning   Just
backward   forward   right

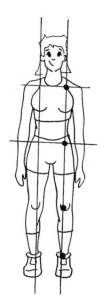

Our major joints are designed to be aligned one on top of the other—the shoulders, hips, knees, ankles, and feet should all line up. One knee, ankle, or hip shouldn't be out to the side or tilted to the side.

Our major joints operate primarily as hinge joints. If they don't line up properly, this puts a torque on them every step we take.

Our joints work best when they are properly aligned

Right side = Left side

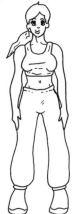

Our bodies are designed to be symmetrical. The right side equals the left. One hip or shoulder shouldn't be more forward or higher than the other. Our weight should be evenly centered on both feet.

Symmetrical

Our pelvis is designed to be upright and not tilted too far forward or back. If it isn't, we start to spill in one direction or the other.

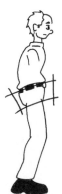
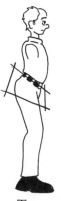
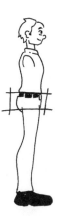

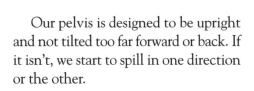

Too far forward

Too far backward

Just right

Our spine is designed to carry our weight with three gentle curves: a slight concave curve in the cervical (neck) region, a slight convex curve in our upper back, and again a slight concave curve or arch in our lower back.

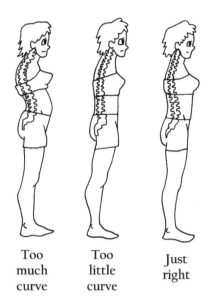

Too much curve   Too little curve   Just right

Alter any of these things and we put ourselves at risk for the downward spiral. Once our alignment is off, the muscles that are stiff become stiffer, and the muscles that are weak become weaker. As a result our alignment or posture deteriorates even further. Pain or simply the disinclination to move leads to further curtailment of movement and further stiffness and weakness. The cycle continues—the downward spiral again.

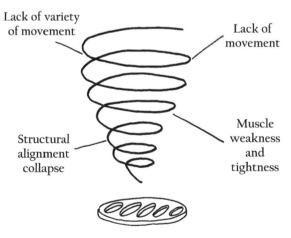

Lack of variety of movement

Lack of movement

Structural alignment collapse

Muscle weakness and tightness

The Downward Spiral Again

> **The key underlying common denominator
> in the downward spiral is our loss of postural alignment.**

That is why the subtitle of this book is "the missing link in health and fitness." Postural alignment is the most frequently overlooked aspect of musculoskeletal health. If you got it, you can do most anything. If you don't "got it," you are in trouble or heading for trouble.

> **Postural malalignment is the hidden
> culprit in our loss of function and our
> musculoskeletal pain and disability.**

Only to the degree that any musculoskeletal fitness plan addresses muscle strength, flexibility, *and* alignment will it succeed long term.

Appearance

You may have picked up this book because you don't like the way you look. You look in the mirror and simply don't like what you see. Your back is rounded or hunched forward; your shoulders are rolled forward; you're slouching, leaning, or collapsing. You look shorter, twisted, or sagging. You look older than you should. You know your posture is off and you want to do something about it.

Our mothers may not have been exactly right on how to correct our posture—there's more to it than just pulling our shoulders back. But they were right on the benefits. With correct posture:

• Others perceive us differently. Like it or not, we are judged and we judge others by their posture. With good posture, we are perceived as more confident, happy, and in control. Older people with correct posture are perceived as younger and sexier.

• We move better. There is a grace and economy of movement that comes with postural alignment.

• We feel better. Our posture, how we stand and move, directly affects our emotions and how we feel.

• All our organ systems work better and more efficiently. Our muscles and bones aren't separate from the rest of our body. A closed chest limits our breathing. A pelvis that is overly tilted forward puts strain on our abdominal organs.

What, Moi?

While some people are aware their posture is off, others may not be quite so aware. Here, right at the beginning, let me warn you:

• It is often very difficult to see one's own malalignment. We are not generally taught what correct alignment is and what exactly to look for. Poor alignment or posture has become visually commonplace; a slouching, casual posture has become vogue. We may look like most everyone else we know. But just because it's common does not make it normal, let alone optimal. You will learn what to look for.

• Your posture or alignment doesn't have to be dramatically off for it to have a considerable effect on your function or to cause pain. Seemingly small distortions in alignment can lead to dramatic alterations in function. And correcting them can lead to equally dramatic returns of function.

• Your alignment may be off and you may not be having any problems at this time because of it. You're lucky—you have a window of opportunity to do something about it now.

• No matter how aberrant our posture may be, it always grows to feel normal and even comfortable to us. So I suggest that even if you do not feel grossly off in posture or alignment that you keep reading.

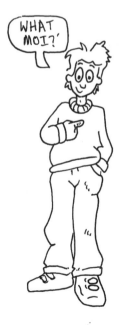

Even if you don't feel your posture is *that* bad, you may be aware of some of the signs and symptoms of faulty posture or alignment. This book is also for you if:

• You have pain in your muscles or joints. If it hurts to do normal things, it shouldn't hurt to do. If you have tendinitis, bursitis, or the early signs of arthritis. Not all pain but a significant amount of muscle and joint pain can be caused by faulty alignment. This encompasses much more pain than we generally think.

• You have reached a plateau in your favorite sport and can go no farther (despite new clubs, rackets or lessons). You suspect it might have something to do with your body but don't know exactly what it is.

• Have cut back on activities. Have cut back or given up your favorite sport or stopped doing physical work or activities you used to enjoy. It just doesn't feel right anymore or you just don't enjoy it as much as you used to. Our bodies often know something is off before we do.

• It's simply taking more effort to go up stairs or do normal things. It worries you that you may be getting old before your time. You don't care about becoming a fitness freak; you just want to be able to comfortably live your normal life.

Or perhaps you see the downward spiral all around you and simply want to maintain maximum function as you grow older, and to prevent the onset of joint, back, and muscle and bone disability as long as you can.

What We Don't Want

Most people don't have the time, luxury, money, or inclination to join a health club or make a concerted physical fitness effort that demands a great deal of their time. We're too busy living our lives.

What we are after is function: something that will improve the quality of our day-to-day living. We want something that will make things easier. We want something that will hold off or postpone the aging process for a few more years while we get our work done.

> Give me something that works
> and doesn't take long to do.

Something that will hold the downward spiral in abeyance for a few more years ... "maybe I'll worry about a total fitness program sometime in the future."

And we want the most bang for our exercise time. If we are going to be required to do something to maintain our function, then don't make us waste time on nonessentials. If you put in ten or twenty or thirty minutes doing something, you want to be pretty darn sure that whatever you're doing is the optimal thing to be doing (or at least pretty near close to it). In a word you don't want to force yourself to slog around some high-school track every morning and end up just as physically dysfunctional as you would have been otherwise. You could have spent that time sleeping.

Posture Alignment answers this need. It works. The exercises require no props or equipment. They can be done at home or in a hotel room when you're on the road—or anywhere.

How Posture Alignment Works

The goal of Posture Alignment is to stretch the muscles that are tight, strengthen the muscles that are weak, and put ourselves back into correct alignment, and then stay that way.

> Whatever functional exercise program you prescribe to, unless it in some way addresses weakness, stiffness, and alignment you won't get long-term results.

The word *posture* comes from the Latin word *ponere*, meaning "to place." But with Posture Alignment we aren't trying to place or hold ourselves in any position. You already know this doesn't work. If you try to hold your shoulders back when they are rolled forward, they won't stay there. After a few seconds they fall back into their same old position. You can't, and your body won't. With Posture Alignment we go after the core muscles groups, release and correct them and make correct posture our home. It becomes the way we stand and move naturally without effort.

We're All Equal

It doesn't matter whether you're old or young, fat or slim. It doesn't matter whether you believe in any of this or not. No esoteric religion or fitness beliefs are necessary. No fitness guru required. It works the same for any and all of us.

When muscles are stretched, we become more flexible. When muscles are used, they become stronger. When our alignment improves, we feel better and are able to move more.

But . . .

This is going to take some effort on your part. After all, it's taken a while to get in this dilemma and it's going to take some time to get out of it (considerably less, however).

We may wish that our bodies were something we could bring in for maintenance at increasingly longer intervals (like today's cars) and forget about the rest of the time. But they're not. Sorry. Like so many other things in life, it's not going to happen and it never will. This is going to take some effort on your part.

No drive-up window. You're going to have to get involved. Get your hands at least a little dirty and all that. It won't require waking-up-at-5:00-A.M.-and-jogging-around-the-track effort, but it will take some effort. And let me guarantee at this point that you will see results. You will be pleasantly surprised. This does work.

However, you are going to have to do two things. You must

- Change the way you think about things a little bit.
- Take some action. Do some exercises to correct or remedy the problem.

Where to begin in all this? Wherever you're at. Anything you do will help.

> Anything you do to move in the direction of improved alignment will help.

While so-called perfect alignment may be a noble goal, anything we do to move ourselves in the direction of improved alignment is of benefit. Any little thing you can do to stave off or hold off your loss of function is worth it. Doing just a few exercises can dramatically improve your appearance and how you feel. A slight change in your alignment may be enough to get rid of a nagging pain. Anything you do—one exercise, one small change in even the way you think about things—can make a difference and allow you to step off the downward spiral.

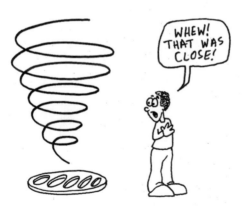

The upcoming chapters discuss in more detail
how and why our bodies need to be correctly
aligned and present the necessary background
for the self-assessment and exercises that follow.

CHAPTER 2

Body Basics

When the human energy field and gravity are
at war, needless to say gravity wins every time.

– Ida Rolf

How does the body work anyway? No, I'm not going to show you pictures of muscles with lots of Latin names. But let's take a walk and find out . . .

The National Museum Of Natural History

Near where I used to live in Washington, D.C. are some of the best museums in the world. One of my favorites is the National Museum of Natural History. As you walk through the exhibits on evolution, you are immediately struck by the similarities in bones and structure between all the prehistoric animals and ourselves.

There are fossils of fish more than 230 million years old with backbones (those bony vertebrae with intervening discs) virtually identical to our own. Dinosaurs share shoulder girdles not unlike our own and have the same humerus and the same paired forearm bones—bones, the same bones, connected by muscles.

The basic elements of our skeletal design have been around for a long time. A very long time. And, one might add, they have been time-tested in a way no consumer product lab could ever do. Designs that weren't up to speed were readily discarded. You might argue that those animals walked on all fours and that our upright posture is somewhat more precarious and prone to injury or not as well developed. Well, continue down the halls of the museum . . .

Depending on current fossil findings, our ancestors began to walk upright about

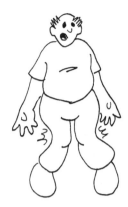

I was just born
with weak knees,
you know.

3.7 million years ago. It is only in the last, say, fifty to one hundred years that we have had the luxury of not physically scraping, clawing, digging, fighting, and wrenching our livelihood from the environment. That 3.7 million years is a long, long time in the consumer product testing lab.

Based on this, it seems reasonable to assume that the design of our body is not flawed. Our knees, backs, shoulders, and wrists are not randomly thrown together. They are sophisticated mechanisms— well thought-out and designed. Has it ever struck you as absurd that we could have evolved over this long period of time and yet be so frail? Wouldn't our species have become extinct long ago if we were *really* so inherently prone to weak knees and ankles, bad backs, and shoulder pain?

To badly paraphrase Shakespeare, the fault doesn't lie with the design of our bodies, it lies with us, with what we are doing (or not doing) with our bodies.

> The design of our body is not flawed.
> It is what we do, or don't do
> that causes the problems.

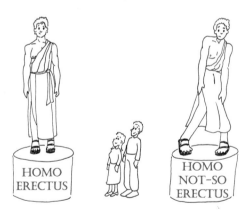

So before we arbitrarily decide, or I might add cavalierly decide, that something is basically wrong with our knees or that they are prone to "fall apart" after a certain age, let's take the opposite viewpoint: something we are doing or not doing is making our knees hurt. Before we are so quick to cut, replace, and generally throw out the model as obsolete, let's consider the opposite. Our strength, flexibility, and alignment have deteriorated which is not allowing our knees to function properly.

> There is no inherent flaw in the design of our bodies.
> Muscular weakness, loss of flexibility,
> and loss of alignment cause the design
> to be unable to function properly.

So what went wrong? If we can assume that our design is not flawed, how did we get out of alignment? I hinted at the answer earlier but let's swing over to the next museum on the Mall, the National Museum of American History, and take a more in-depth look . . .

Civilization

It's actually quite simple. You already know the answer to what went wrong. We don't move enough. And when we do move, we move in the same repetitive ways, never utilizing our full range of movements and rarely requiring strength from all of our muscles. Certain muscles, our sitting and walking muscles for example, get lots of stimulation; other muscles are underutilized. Because certain muscles get strong and certain muscles get weak, we lose correct alignment. We stop being a balanced whole.

Sure, there is a lot of activity going on in our lives, a lot of busy-ness. But for most people it entails a lot of sitting and driving. We don't do all the physical things we used to have to do to wrench out a living. We don't perform the movements and activities that were once the mainstay of our survival as a species. And like everything else, when something isn't used, the ability becomes lost or in this case, quiescent. You've heard this before, but I'll say it again.

> We don't move enough. We don't move in
> varied enough ways. And because of that
> certain functions have become quiescent
> and our alignment has fallen apart.

To be fair, this isn't entirely our fault. *Society no longer requires that we move as much.* Technology has made it easier and easier to get by with moving less and less. In fact, sometimes the whole goal of the ergonomic movement seems to be to make everything so inanely simple to operate and at such a convenient waist-high level that we never need to lean or stretch to reach anything, let alone use any significant strength. Perhaps we could all rest comfortably in cushy, back-supported chairs all day and control our worlds with the click of a mouse or a remote control. It sounds like a futuristic dream, or a nightmare.

However, the fact remains that, despite our intelligence and great technological advances, we are and will remain—one hesitates to say it—animals. And just as plants need light to thrive, just as machinery needs lubrication to keep operating properly, we need functional movement to maintain the health of these bodies.

Look at some of the turn-of-the-century tools in the National Museum of American History or look at something like the 1902 Sears Roebuck catalog. One hundred years ago everything was heavier and demanded far more physical strength to operate. Everything required turning, screwing, clipping, pulling, yanking, pushing, grinding, pounding (no nail guns), or hitching. In the kitchen it was grinding, grating, skinning, beating, kneading, sewing, cutting. At work it was swinging, raking, shoveling, lifting, hauling . . . well, you get the idea. It's interesting that so many devices required turning something by using the hands and shoulders. Now the only things I can readily think of that requires a similar movement are a manual can opener and the roll-up windows in cars—both of which are becoming virtually obsolete.

A great deal of varied physical effort was required for our ancestors just to get from dawn to dusk. But for us everyday things get physically easier and easier. There are more and more things that make us less prone to move. There are more escalators, elevators, and moving walkways where there used to be stairs. There are food processors where there used to be knives, graters, and mixing bowls. There are weed wackers where there used to be hand-operated clippers. Everything gets physically easier and easier and less demanding until one fears it will soon reach an inane level of physical simplicity—almost like television.

> Society in general no longer supports
> or requires varied and functional movement.
> And it keeps getting worse.

Devices invented as aids to help people—to make things easier and go faster—now threaten our existence. Things that used to be luxuries have now become necessities. More and more people are now *no longer able* to go up and down multiple flights of stairs or to open a heavy door. And it's happening at younger and younger ages. We are fast becoming a nation of the physically disabled.

> If we aren't careful, technology conspires
> to make us weaker and weaker.

I am not against technology or making things easier and by no means do I want to go back to earlier times. I'm all for labor-saving devices as much as the next guy. But if we aren't aware of this trend and if we don't do something to counteract it in our individual lives, we're in trouble.

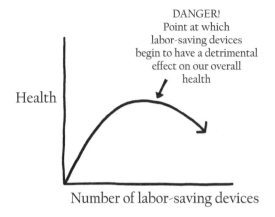

Number of labor-saving devices

If you drew a graph of all this, it might look something like this. There would reach a point where all the labor-saving devices and all the lack of movement and lifting would start to have a detrimental effect.

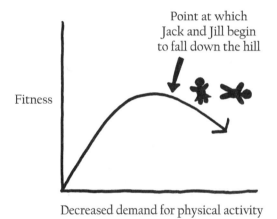

Decreased demand for physical activity

A graph could be drawn for each of us as individuals also. There reaches a point where Jack and Jill begin to fall down the hill.

We're Smart Not To

Actually, it is our cleverness and survivability as a species that makes us not want to do any more than we have to. Why walk when you can ride? Why stand when you can sit? We aren't really lazy. Why walk when you can ride is a smart evolutionary thing when it comes to conserving energy. It makes sense not to move or do any more than we have to.

Even any form of "exercise" goes against this innate grain. It *is* purposeless movement and activity. Why not just stay back in the cave until the time comes when we need to do something. And lots of people do exactly that.

This is why it takes effort to exercise. It has to feel like an effort because it is. Now more than ever, for most of us, it has become necessary to do *something* just to maintain a baseline level of fitness in order to prevent that ride down the spiral.

We have reached the point where, now more than ever, supplemental or remedial activity is necessary to maintain our function.

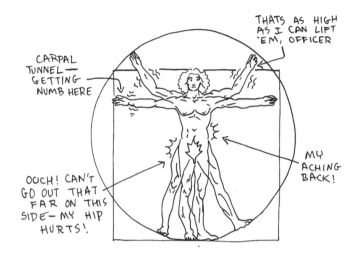

Newton's Laws

No, these aren't really Newton's laws but they just as well might be. Let's call them Newton's Laws of Movement.

- Those who move tend to keep moving. Those who move less and less tend to come to a stop.
- Those who move in varied ways retain the ability to move in varied ways.

The G-Word

Gravity: the G-word. Until the day we die, this force rains down on us from above. On the just and the unjust. It is our constant, relentless companion. It never sleeps.

Pretend you were a ball of Silly Putty®. Left to its own devices, gravity over time would leave you puddled on the ground.

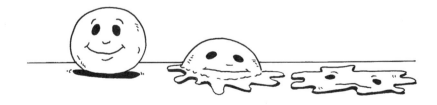

It is no different with our bodies. Gravity is constantly pushing down from above. Any place we don't hold ourselves up, gravity wins.

> ## Until the day we die, we carry on a constant battle with gravity.

Or imagine yourself in a wind tunnel, one of those tunnels where they test cars and other objects for aerodynamic stability. You're standing in the wind tunnel and the wind from the big fan at the end is blowing in your face and ruffling your clothing. If you stick your hand out, the wind grabs at it and attempts to force it backward.

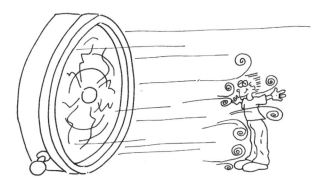

Now, close your eyes while we rotate the big wind tunnel fan ninety degrees and put it on the ceiling so that the wind is coming at you from above. Gravity is a vertical vector force.

If your body is standing straight and tall, the wind from above easily splits and passes on all sides of you. But lean your head forward a little and you will feel the wind forcing down on the back of your neck. Stick your bottom out a little and you will feel the wind attempt to take hold and force you to the ground.

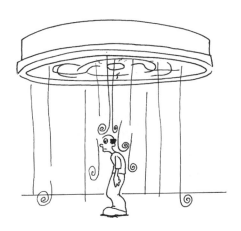

The only difference between gravity and our wind tunnel example is that gravity is silent. It doesn't make all those blowing noises and hence we tend to forget it's there. *And it is never turned off.*

What holds us up against this interminable force called gravity anyway? Our skeleton? Our bones? Nope. If you look back at all the skeletons in the Museum of Natural History, you'll notice all the bones are wired together and held up by metal rods. Bones *are* important, but the correct answer is our muscles. Our muscles hold us upright. And if our muscles don't hold us up then we start to move closer and closer and closer to the ground. That's where we are all going eventually, but we don't want to go there before our time.

Let's go back to our vertical wind tunnel example once more. Once we deviate from our vertical alignment, once we stick any body part out into the windstream, it requires muscular effort and strain to hold it there.

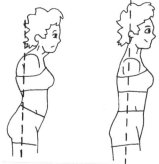

Head forward   Healthy in-line head position

It is the same with the vertical alignment of our bodies. Suppose, for example, our head is too far forward of our body, something that is commonly seen. It takes muscular effort and strain to hold it out there. Gravity wants to get a hold of it and push it down, and we have to hold it up.

And those muscles that hold our head there often become tired or go into spasm. They weren't designed to continuously hold our big heads (15 pounds!) out at an angle. If they are required to, they get worn out and tired. If you're chronically hunched over a computer or a desk, you have good reason to feel stress, strain, and tension in your neck, upper back, and shoulders. You should.

It is the same if we chronically lean forward, backward, or to the side. We have to use muscular effort to hold ourselves there. Aligning our posture produces increased energy in part by curtailing these unnecessary expenditures of energy.

> When we are not aligned with gravity, it produces undo strain and tension on joints and muscles and we expend additional amounts of energy to stay upright.

So far we've described gravity as a somewhat evil companion who is always trying to bring us down. But there is another side to gravity. Gravity provides a constant load to our muscles and bones which keeps them strong to fight against . . . gravity. One of the problems with weightlessness in space travel (the National Air and Space Museum is right across the Mall but we won't go there) is that astronauts quickly lose their load-bearing muscle mass and strength.

But let's return back to the Museum of American History . . .

Physics, Engineering, and Architecture

On the lower level of the museum there are exhibits on construction and bridge building. For a building to stand, it must be aligned with gravity. There's that G-word again. If you look around, you'll notice that all buildings are upright, that is, they are vertically aligned with gravity. Ones that can't maintain this verticality (the Leaning Tower of Pisa being one notable exception) are generally hauled away in dump trucks.

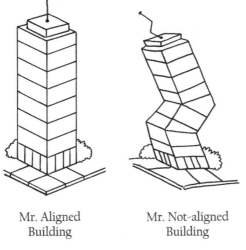

Mr. Aligned
Building

Mr. Not-aligned
Building

No competent builder would build a building with one part leaning way out without adequate support. That would produce inordinate amounts of stress on the supporting structure and eventually it would fail.

Our bodies instinctively know this too. If our head, for example, is leaned too far forward, we adjust our hips and backs to compensate in an attempt to re-align ourselves with gravity.

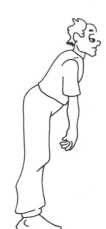

Head and body
leaned forward

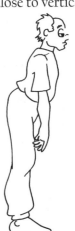

Compensation to
bring body back
close to vertical

> When our alignment becomes
> distorted, our bodies compensate
> in various ways to stay balanced.

But this compensation has problems. It would be as if a builder, instead of fixing the primary problem, simply shifted a section of the building over several yards to accommodate for it. Not a good idea for buildings; not a good idea for our bodies.

Compensation in one area leads to increased strain in another area, which leads to further compensation to handle that, which leads to increased strain somewhere else. Our old friend, the downward spiral occurs again—an increasing cascade of detrimental effects because the real problem was never addressed.

> Malalignment with gravity leads to strain,
> which leads to compensation, which leads to
> strain in other areas and further compensation.

Let's leave the museums and look at a flexible box . . .

A Flexible Box

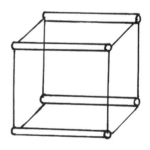

Imagine a box made out of sticks and wire—two sticks at the top and two at the bottom held in place by flexible metal wires.

When you push on one corner of the flexible box, the other corners change position also. Because the stiff sections can't bend to any great degree, the entire structure has to twist slightly, by going either forward, backward, up, or down, but they can't stay in the same place. A scientist might describe this by saying that if the structure becomes altered in one plane, it cannot yield in another plane without twisting.

Here are some of the strange permutations we can make with our box by pulling, pushing, lifting, or dropping one of the corners.

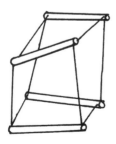
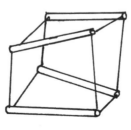
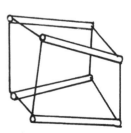

The human body is like our flexible box. Our bones are like the sticks and the muscles, ligaments, tendons, and other connective tissues are like the flexible metal wires. The top of the box is our shoulder girdle; the bottom of the box is our pelvis.

If one shoulder is held or lifted higher than the other, by definition it *has to* cause an alteration in the alignment or strain in the other shoulder and in our pelvis. If one side of our pelvis is more forward or higher than the other, it *has to* cause an alteration in the alignment or strain in the other side and in our houlders.

Try leaning one of your shoulders slightly forward. If you concentrate closely, you immediately feel a corresponding movement in the hip on the same side while the opposite shoulder and hip move backward.

> Our shoulders and hips form a flexible box.
> If one part is out of alignment, by definition
> the other parts must be also.

Healthy
shoulder
box

Altered
shoulder
box

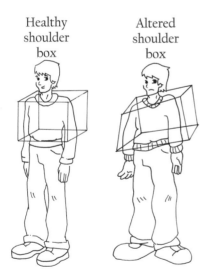

People often become frozen in one of these altered box positions. It need not be as dramatic as in the illustration; often it is much more subtle. But any asymmetry of shoulder and hip alignment can lead to strain or pain in one or both shoulders or hips.

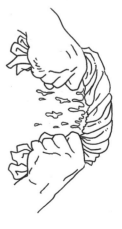

Another way of looking at this is to think of it as a rotational abnormality. The body is twisted slightly around its axis—one part goes forward while another part goes back—like holding a towel in your hand and twisting it.

No matter which analogy you use, it is important that we correct this altered box position or twist. In Posture Alignment, we often have to work on areas distant from the problem to correct them. It might not initially make sense to do an exercise for you hips if your shoulders are out of line. But your shoulders can only come back into alignment to the extent that your hips come back into alignment.

> With Posture Alignment, we often have to work on tightness or weakness in an area distant from the problem before it will correct itself.

And this can't happen all at once; it occurs over time. The muscles that hold the hips out of alignment let go a little, which allows the shoulders to move back slightly, which allows the hips to move back a little more toward correct alignment.

> Our bodies are integrated wholes. If one part is out of line, other parts must be out of line. For one part to get back into position often another part distant from it has to move first.

This is the reason that if your shoulders are rolled forward you can pull them back until you are blue in the face but they won't stay there. And it's also the reason many of our other attempts to correct our posture may not have worked.

Often until one piece of the puzzle distant from the area of concern is unlocked and released, another piece can't be brought back into alignment.

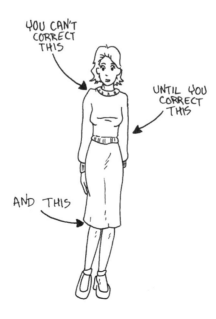

This is also why many people can't get the flexibility they want despite their persistent efforts. I was a victim of this. In a yoga class, I struggled to get one of my hips to open up. At home I would place a fifty-pound bag of concrete on one of my thighs (I don't recommend this) to try to get it to relax and flop down. It never would. It couldn't. Until some deeper muscles were released and realigned, access was denied.

The pelvis is the pivotal controlling area of the body. As the pelvis is aligned, so goes the rest of the body (see ITPS: "It's the Pelvis, Silly" in Chapter 4). The second key area is the shoulders.

You remember the song, "the hip bone's connected to the knee bone, the knee bone's connected to the . . ." well it all comes back to the pelvis and the shoulders.

Our Bodies As Dynamic Structures

One of the big differences between, say, something like a building and a human being is that if a building tips over or gets bent out of shape, it can't fix itself. All the elements in a building are static, that is, they remain the same.

The human body is different. Not only do our bodies have the ability to right themselves but they have the ability to change shape, to adapt. We have the ability to get out of postural alignment and to get back into it.

> Our bodies are dynamic structures.
> They have the ability to get back into shape.

Function creates structure is an old maxim of the natural sciences. This simply means that the demands placed on a living creature determine the shape it has to take to adapt to them.

This is true in evolutionary terms where over time, millions of years, environmental stress and strain led to us looking the way we look. And it is also true for us and other animals in everyday terms such as where the demand for a squirrel to climb up a tree maintains the muscles and structural alignment necessary for it to do that.

Wolff's Law

In 1892, a man named Julius Wolff postulated a number of laws related to bone. He basically said that bone adapts both its external form and internal structure to the loads exerted on it. Simply put, bone changes its shape and strength based on how much load is placed on it. That is, bone changes depending on where it is pulled on or pushed on over periods of time.

This is the reason broken bones heal, bone spurs occur, and ugly little bony protrusions called osteophytes are present on some people's X rays. Bone like everything else in our bodies adapts to the stress and strain placed on it. And this is why the effects of osteoporosis can be mitigated to some degree by weight-lifting programs, which may allow new bone to be laid down.

What's true for bone is also true to a greater degree for muscle. Muscle adapts and develops increased strength based on the loads placed on it. We all know this. If you lift weights, the muscles you use get stronger.

It is also true for ligaments and tendons. They adapt to and respond to the loads placed on them, becoming stronger and more resilient.

> Bones, muscles, ligaments, and tendons adapt
> and get stronger based on the load placed on them.

Unfortunately, the opposite is also true. If not used, if not enough load or demand is placed on bone, muscles, ligaments, and tendons, they lose their strength.

Immobilization

Some of the most disconcerting research you can read is on the effects of being bedridden or immobilized for any period of time. If you've ever been sick in bed or had a cast on for any length of time, you know this. When you recover even simple things like getting up to brush your teeth or taking a few steps can be overwhelmingly hard.

We all know this intuitively but here are the facts about immobilization.

• Causes loss of muscle mass and strength. With immobilization, loss of strength occurs at 1-1.5 % per day. With immobilization in a plaster cast, you lose 22% of your strength in the first seven days!

• Leads to reduced extensibility of muscle tissues. They grow more rigid.

• Leads to loss of bone density and strength.

• Causes all connective tissue (joint tissue, tendons, ligaments, and fascia) to lose their elasticity due to actual chemical changes in structure.

• Leads to reduced function and efficiency of all major organ systems of the body: circulatory, respiratory, digestive, and endocrine.

And the really disconcerting fact is that it takes a long time to recover from this degeneration and return to normal. Often it takes years. Doctors and hospitals are now aware of this, which is one of the reasons they encourage early mobilization for almost all injuries and surgeries.

So why am I talking about immobilization. One reason might be to encourage you to avoid being immobilized. If you're hurt or sick, try to get up and get moving as soon as possible.

The other reason is that a sedentary lifestyle or a lifestyle where we don't move all our parts immobilizes us. To a greater or lesser degree, we experience similar declines in function. Under-utilized areas of the body undergo similar immobilization effects. The bones that aren't stressed lose mineral content and strength. The muscles we don't use lose strength and become more rigid. The joints we don't move become tighter and less flexible.

> Lack of demand placed on bones, muscles, ligaments, and tendons leads to loss of function.

Aging

I sort of side-slipped the aging question earlier by saying it didn't matter. It doesn't matter because there is nothing we can do about the fixed parameters of aging, although there is still considerable debate on what those parameters are.

In any case, the facts on aging—after age 35 or so—are also a bit disconcerting. They are almost a graduated form of the immobilization facts. Here are a few of the facts on aging.

• There is a gradual automatic loss of muscle mass and strength. If you don't do anything to prevent it, you automatically lose 5-7 pounds of muscle mass every decade. Muscle mass is also the prime determinant of resting metabolic rate. With loss of muscle mass, resting metabolic rate decreases. It gets easier to get fat!

• There is a gradual loss of bone mineral density and bone strength with a particularly dramatic drop-off for women after menopause.

• Connective tissue loses water content and becomes increasingly rigid.

The facts on aging are not in our favor. We are fighting an uphill battle.

The 1996 Surgeon General's Report on Physical Activity and Health (USDHHS 1996) made an interesting observation ". . . disuse syndromes closely resemble age-related changes in many organ systems." This includes the musculoskeletal system. What this is saying is that disuse to a large extent equals aging.

> Disuse to a large extent equals aging.

The report goes on to say that resumption of activity can reverse many of these effects. Many people, however, experience a double-whammy effect; the biological effects of aging combined with an increasingly sedentary lifestyle accelerate the downward spiral.

Functional Reserve

The ability of a given organ system to withstand the demands placed on it is termed its functional reserve.

If any of our organ systems are working at their maximum to begin with, they often cannot take the additional strain of any further compromise in their function. This is what causes the elderly to be more prone to sickness and to complications when they do get sick. A "bad cold" turns into pneumonia. Additional demand on an already fully-taxed heart precipitates heart failure. And this is what eventually causes us all to die; we eventually have no functional reserve left to combat an overwhelming threat.

It is the same with the musculoskeletal system. If our muscles are working at their maximum every day just to maintain us, there is nothing left if any additional demand is placed on them. If we are suddenly required to do anything outside our normal routine, we pull a muscle or injure a joint. If we trip, we don't have the additional muscular strength and balance to catch ourselves. If we are suddenly demanded to bend or reach too far behind ourselves, we don't have the flexibility to do it, and we get hurt.

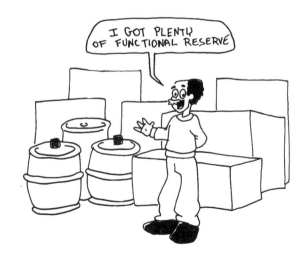

One of the goals of Posture Alignment is to build up reserves in our strength and flexibility so that whatever happens we won't be so easily overwhelmed by it, both on a day-to-day and a long-term basis.

What You Need To Know About Muscles

In simplest terms, muscles work in pairs or teams. For every muscle on the front of your body, there is one on the back of your body that does the same thing in the opposite direction. And for every muscle on one side of your body, there is one like it on the opposite side of your body.

Because of the shape of the body, the muscles on front or back, for example, may not look the same. The one that pulls a bone to the front may be short and fan-shaped; the one that pulls the same bone backward may be long and narrow.

The fancy names for these muscle pairs are agonists and antagonists. In simplest terms, for us to move a joint, the muscle on one side of it (the agonist) contracts, while the muscle on the other side (the antagonist) relaxes. And the bone they control changes its position in space. Agonist and antagonist sound so adversarial; perhaps it is better to think of them as cooperating teams of muscles.

> Muscles work in cooperating teams.

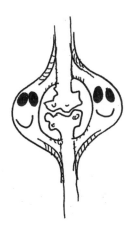

Now think of a muscle pair on either side of a joint. One muscle is on the right side, the other on the left side. In the optimal situation, both are evenly balanced with respect to length and strength, and the joint is held in equilibrium, that is, with no unnecessary compression or tension on either side.

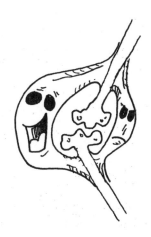

Now think of the same joint if one muscle is overdeveloped, if it is tighter and stronger than its partner. Our picture would look like this.

We commonly see this in the weight lifter who has overdeveloped his biceps at the expense of his triceps. He walks around with his arms bent because one muscle is more developed than the other.

But don't think you are immune just because you don't lift weights. This occurs to greater or lesser degrees in all of us. Our posture in fact is a composite picture of all these muscles, some too tight, some too weak, and some just right.

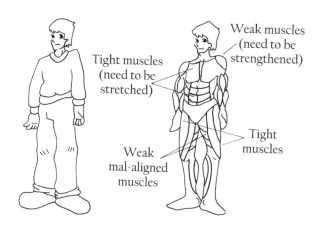

For each one of us we could draw a similar picture. And you can begin to see that it is not just a matter of getting stronger. Posture Alignment is about bringing balance and alignment to the body's structure by making the tight areas more flexible and the weak areas stronger so that things line up as they should.

Each muscle also has an optimal length and angle where it works the best. Just as a pulley wouldn't function properly if its parts aren't lined up, each muscle does its best work when it is aligned as it should be. Muscles can often somehow get the job done even when they're not in the correct alignment, but they are definitely not as happy as they could be.

> Every muscle has an optimal alignment
> where it is most happy and efficient.

No Muscle Is An Island

While it is useful and convenient to talk of individual muscles and their functions, truly speaking we don't move or function that way. Even our most simple everyday movements are far more complex, requiring many muscles to work in harmony by contracting and releasing in a coordinated manner. That's why isolating and developing a single muscle isn't always the best idea, since the other muscles, large and small, that must work in concert with it, aren't being trained along with it.

Rather than list all the muscles involved, it makes more sense to simply say, "the muscles that allow us to get up off a chair and reach forward to pick something up."

What You Need To Know About Joints

Knees, ankles, shoulders, hips—now that's where our problems are. That's where we hurt, not in our muscles. But if you go back to the picture of our pair of muscles around a joint, you see that it is the muscles that determine the joint's position. It is the alignment and balance of the muscles surrounding a joint that determine whether stress, strain, or grinding is going to occur in the joint. If the muscle on one side of a joint is too strong, the joint will be slightly cock-eyed, tilted, or rotated slightly. This alters the compression and tension on the joint—more pressure is being put on one area of the joint's articular surface than other areas. This also causes strain on the ligaments surrounding the joint. It may also lead to destruction of cartilage, bursitis, or tendonitis along with an increased propensity to injury because of the altered alignment.

And if your joints aren't lined up right, you cannot walk or run, sit down and stand up as effectively as you might.

> Imbalanced muscles lead to distortion of joint alignment and abnormal compression and strain on the joint itself.

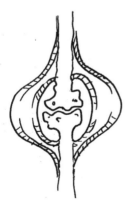

Muscles need
to be balanced
on both sides
of a joint

Scientific analyses of joints have defined the alignment where joint surfaces are optimally meant to carry weight. Often only a few degrees of torque or malalignment are enough to drastically alter the compression and tension on a joint.

Joint pain is often a sign of what is going
on with the strength and alignment of
the muscles surrounding a joint.

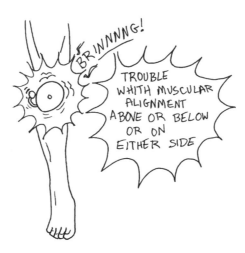

Joint malalignment is a timebomb waiting to go off. Joint malalignment leads to pain or disability, which leads to moving less, which leads to key muscles becoming weaker still. Malalignment worsens; joints hurt more and move less. The cycle continues.

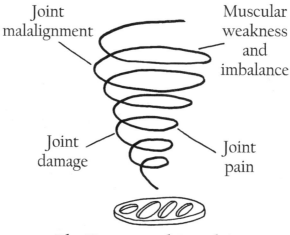

The Downward Spiral Again

Flexibility

Why do we want flexibility? Because we gotta move. Because we have to reach down to pick things up. Because we've got to reach up to put things away. Because we have to get from here to there, to hit a baseball and to pirouette.

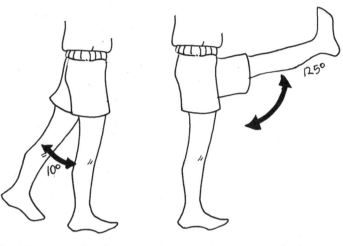

Range of motion refers to the degrees of arc each of our joints can circumscribe. For example, the normal range of motion at the hip joint is 10 degrees of extension (bending it backward) and 125 degrees of flexion (bending it forward).

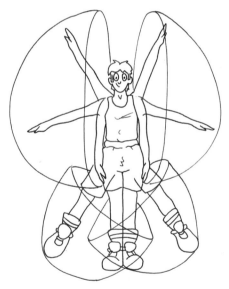

For many of our joints, notably our hips and shoulders, the ranges of motion extend in multiple planes describing 3-D ranges through which they can comfortably move.

But as stated before, often as we get older, as our alignment gets off, as we move less and less, our range of motion (the arcs we can comfortably move our joints through) becomes less and less. What used to be comfortable to do such as reaching way above our heads or checking the blind spot while driving now becomes harder to do.

Posture Alignment is concerned with maintaining maximum range of motion. No, you don't have to be able to twist into a pretzel, but like the life raft example in the first chapter, you don't want to concede your range of motion and flexibility before its time.

> ## We want to maximize and maintain
> ## our joints' ranges of motion.

We also want our joints to hang out, to reside, somewhere in the middle of their ranges of motion. We don't want them maxed out to either extreme. That is, you don't want a knee or ankle chronically flared way out to the side so that the ligaments surrounding the knee or ankle are stretched to the max.

If a joint is chronically twisted or tilted so that it is at the extreme of its movement range, any requirement for it to move any farther in that direction will cause something to break, snap, or tear. A joint residing in the maxed-out position puts undo stress on muscles, tendons, and ligaments. There is no room for play, literally and figuratively. The joint becomes an accident waiting to happen.

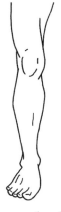

Foot and ankle
in healthy in-line
position with
no excessive
strain

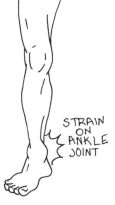

Foot and ankle
overly everted
to one side

A healthy, balanced joint is like a tennis player in the ready position. She is neither leaning too far forward or back, or too far to one side or the other. Wherever the ball comes from, she is ready and able to move in that direction.

> ## We want our joints to reside in the
> ## middle of their ranges of motion.

Where We're Going With All This

Here is a quick, close approximation of what optimal posture should look and feel like:

• Stand with your feet hip-width apart, next to a large floor-length mirror if possible.

• Turn both feet inward so that your toes touch while your heels remain separated about eight inches apart (pigeon-toed).

• Gently straighten your legs as much as possible. You should feel your pelvis lift up and a slight stretch across the front of your groins.

• Now lift your shoulders up and then back, and then let them relax downward.

This posture (aside from your feet) gives a very close approximation of correct anatomical alignment. Look at yourself in the mirror and see how you feel. You may have gained a good two inches in height and feel increased energy and poise. This is how you are supposed to look. This is where we are going.

So let's put this all together and
take a closer look at two people,
Bob and Dave, and see why they move
and stand and walk differently.

CHAPTER 3

Why Bob Doesn't Look
Or Move Like Dave

The form of the body is the result
of the sum of its everyday movements.

– Bess Mensendick

Imagine yourself at a typical driving range. A row of amateur golfers are lined up taking swings at the ball. Each one has their own peculiar way of hitting the ball. One wags his hips this way, one wags the other way. One shifts her weight back, one forward. One lifts a shoulder, one drops it. Each has his or her own way of getting the job done—in this case getting a golf ball to go in the general direction of down a fairway.

Why do they do this differently? Simply habit or lack of training? Perhaps.

Now let's take a closer look at two guys, Bob and Dave. They could just as easily be two women, Rita or Darlene, or a man and a woman. Despite any social inequalities, when it comes to postural alignment and which muscles need to be used to do a given job, men and women are exactly the same. Man equals woman and woman equals man in body alignment and functional anatomy.

When Bob gets down on the floor and gets up, it looks different than when Dave does the same thing. Bob uses his hands to push to the side and then hoists himself up shifting his weight forward and pressing his hands against his thighs. Dave gets up by leaning to one side, swinging one leg beneath him and then rising up.

Why do they do this differently?

And for that matter once they are standing up, why is Bob's posture different from Dave's posture? Bob's right shoulder is lifted slightly and one foot is pointing more out to the side than the other. Dave stands with one foot (his left) pointing way out to the side and his hips rolled backward almost as if he is sitting in a chair even when he is standing.

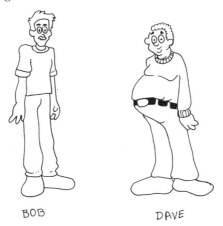

BOB   DAVE

The most common answer and the one most people would be comfortable with is that Dave is different from Bob, that is, their bodies are different. That's just the way they are. You know, genetics and all that. Or maybe they have different habits. Or perhaps we're seeing the results of aging (there's that word again) in one and not in the other.

All the above answers are true. But the real answer underlying all of these since the only thing that puts bones where they are or moves them is *muscles*. Bob is using different muscles and different groups of muscles than Dave is. To be more precise, Dave and Bob have the same sets of muscles. However, different ones are weak, strong, tight, or loose relative to each other causing them both to stand and be balanced in different ways with respect to gravity. Bob and Dave stand and move differently to accommodate their relative weaknesses and strengths just as our golfers did.

If you took composite pictures of Bob and Dave, you might be able to label certain muscle groups as being either too tight, too weak, or just right.

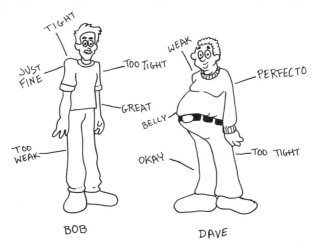

BOB   DAVE

This would give you a composite view of exactly what is going on and explain their different ways of standing and of doing things. It would explain the different ways they *need* to do things.

> Muscular imbalances (some muscles too tight,
> too weak, or too strong) are what cause our
> differences in posture and movement

Why There Really Is No Such Thing As Bad Posture

What? Of course, there's bad posture. That's what this book is about, isn't it?

No, sorry. There *really* is no such thing as bad posture because how we each stand and move is a perfect, composite representation of the habitual demands and stimuli placed on our bodies. It has to be that way. Everybody's body tells their individual story.

> The way you stand and move perfectly represents
> the areas of tight, loose, weak, and strong muscles
> and the amount and type of stimulus you have
> given your body and are giving it now.

And it follows from this: if we change the amount and type of stimulus placed on our bodies, our posture will change.

How did it get this way anyway? I mean, why aren't we all the same? Don't we all get basically the same stimulation? And some of us exercise—Bob runs and Dave plays tennis, you know . . .

The Great Improviser

Our bodies are great improvisers. They make due with what is available. That is why we have survived for so long.

Let's play a game for a minute. Imagine I put a splint on your right knee so that you can't bend it, and then ask you to walk. Can you do it? Sure. You'd simply walk with that leg straight. You can't bend your knee so you'd simply lift your right hip higher and swing your leg around to propel yourself forward.

But now what if I added something else? What if I put a hard object, let's say a marble, in the bottom heel portion of your left shoe making it uncomfortable to put weight there. Could you still walk? No problemo. You'd continue walking with your right leg straight while lifting up your left heel so that when you walk you won't come down on that area.

Now I put a brace on your back so that your right shoulder is tilted forward and down . . . well, you get the idea. For virtually anything I do, you and your body will automatically come up with a solution, working around the areas of limitation (the splint), and avoiding the areas that cause discomfort (the marble). Through some permutation or combination of movements you will get the job done.

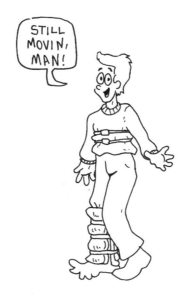

In real life this is what is going on to greater or lesser degrees with our bodies. Things have happened and we have compensated for them. We don't have visible splints but we have developed similar areas of tightness and contraction and compensatory movements for them. Most often our "splints" don't come on immediately as in the example but instead occur over time. And hence our compensations evolve over time also.

How do we get these imbalances? We acquire them. Just as through our upbringing and life experiences we acquire our character, through the physical experiences of our lives, our bodies acquire their character.

How We Get That Way

Let's pretend for a moment that we all start out functional, that is, with everything all lined up and every muscle, bone, ligament, and tendon doing their job—the ideal man or woman.

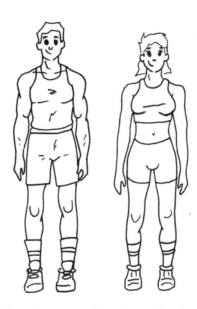

But wait a minute. Then because of work or school we are not as active as we were before. From sitting so much, the muscles in our legs get lazy while other muscles, the muscles that bend our pelvis forward at our hips with sitting, get tight. We do this for months, years. We have just acquired an imbalance.

Then let's say we get hurt. We fracture our ankle and it is in a cast for a month. As in the example above, we don't use the same muscles we did to walk, and when the cast is removed, we walk with our foot just slightly cocked to one side. Those muscles that we should use to walk on that side aren't quite up to snuff. And maybe we acquire a little tilt to the way we walk.

We do one sport to the exclusion of all others. The muscles needed to do that sport grow strong while other muscles that we don't regularly use grow weak and veritably fall by the wayside.

We work a lot at the office. We have a desk chair that we love. Although extremely comfortable, it tilts our spine too far back. We spend long hours sitting there working.

We never reach up over our heads or only on a rare occasion to put in a light bulb. The muscles required to lift our arms grow weak. We lose flexibility in our shoulders.

We carry a heavy purse always over our right shoulder or a briefcase always in our left hand. We carry our baby on our right hip. We swing our tennis racket with our right hand. Our weight and balance end up being more on one foot than the other.

And we imitate our parents, friends, or TV or movie idols—the way they stand, move, and gesture.

Any and all of these things (I'm sure you can come up with some more) can lead to muscle imbalances, front to back, side to side. The fact is . . .

> ## We're always exercising.

You might think that these are little things are inconsequential. Do all these little things make a difference? Yes! All these little habits given enough time like erosion—months, years, decades—become firmly fixed and entrenched in our musculoskeletal psyche.

And our bodies automatically compensate for these muscular imbalances. If one muscle is weak, another one often takes over for it—one that is not be designed to do the job. For example, if the muscles on one side are weak and lazy, other muscles end up carrying an additional burden. But those muscles that stepped in to do the job, *that ain't their job!*

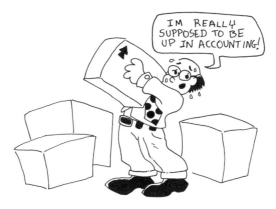

And it's not long before these helping muscles become over-stressed and frazzled, which leads to more problems. What starts off as the body's attempt to compensate for weakness in one area results in too much work or stress in another area. Like a pocket puzzle, the more pieces we move the more out of line things get.

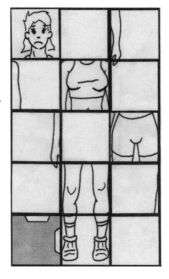
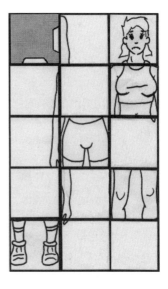

See, the problem with improvisation or compensation is that it is just that, a temporary fix. It wasn't meant to become permanent. You can walk with your leg straight but eventually it will make you unbalanced. The muscles that lift your hip on that side will get stronger than those on the other side. You will lean to one side. Everything will be thrown out of whack. And it's the same with any other asymmetry or imbalance.

Can you see the pattern here? One thing gets out of whack and it leads to a whole cascade of other things getting out of line. The end result is a change in our posture—the way we walk and the way we look when we stand in front of the mirror. To repeat what I said earlier in another way . . .

> Your body, my body, everybody's body tells
> the composite story of all the stresses placed
> on it and all the subsequent improvisations
> and compensations for those stresses.

Then we may decide to exercise! If we aren't careful this either perpetuates or throws another level of dysfunction into the soup. Our dysfunctions can grow worse. By nature, we tend to use the already-strong muscles. The strong muscles get stronger and the weak muscles, well . . . they get weaker. We simply mold our bodies into a more solidified version of ourselves.

Going back to our two fellows. . . remember one of Bob's shoulders being higher than the other and one foot pointing more out to the side. By now you know that this means certain groups of muscles are tighter and stronger on one side and weaker and more stretched on the other.

But now when Bob exercises, when he lifts weights let's say, if he isn't careful he will tend to reinforce the positioning of the already-tight muscles. Bob feels he is getting fit. In certain ways he is. He can lift more. But he is also making himself into a more-firmly entrenched version of Bob.

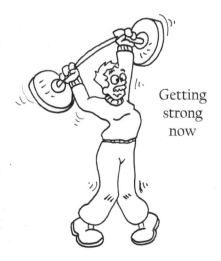

Getting
strong
now

We often tend not to do the exercises that would isolate our weak muscles, or we do them in ways that "cheat," again allowing the already-strong muscles to carry the load of doing an exercise. Not liking an exercise, or when an exercise is "hard," most often means it's an exercise we need to do and can't cheat at (more on this in Chapter 5).

> **The Tailor Story**
> A man goes to a tailor to have a suit designed and constructed. The finished suit is all wrong; it's too long in one leg, bunched up in the back, and one sleeve is way below his fingers. Instead of correctly altering the suit, the tailor tells the man to drop one shoulder. That immediately makes the sleeve the right length. He then tells the man to hunch forward slightly. That takes care of the bunching in the back. And by walking with a bent knee, the trouser leg suddenly becomes the proper length.
>
> This is exactly what we do with our compensations. Instead of fixing the root of the problem, we often make adjustments and compensations that make things worse.

Why You Can't Do It

Have you ever seen one of those TV shows where ultra-fit trainers are trying to coax a bunch of overweight businessmen over a wall or through an Outward Bound-type rope course?

There is invariably one participant who can't make it over the wall and the trainer cajoles them like a drill instructor, "Come on! You can do it!" I certainly understand the idea of pushing ourselves or the value of having others push us beyond our perceived limits. But often the reason this man or woman can't make it over the wall has nothing to do with drive or will-power. In fact, one might even suspect that these business leaders have more drive and willpower than the trainers!

The reason the participant can't make it over the wall is because the muscles required to do that are weak or virtually non-existent. It would be akin to asking the outdoor trainer to rework the inventory or set the budget for the next fiscal quarter. You could coax or prod him forward all you want, "Come on, you can do it! Come on now!" But it ain't going to happen.

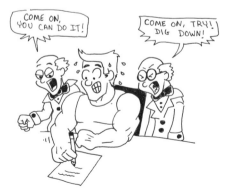

> If you can't do something, there is nothing
> wrong with you. Certain muscles have just
> gotten weak or tight. When you stretch the shortened
> muscles and strengthen the weak muscles,
> you will be able to do it.

For some people some of their muscles have gotten very weak from lack of use—not just plain-old-ordinary weak but crawled-into-a-ball-and-gone-to-sleep weak. They haven't been doing their job and they have no intention of doing their job, thank you very much.

Our Bodies Know What's Going On

Let's fast forward the tape and now we find Bob and Dave standing on the edge of a small ravine. Dave easily jumps across and then turns back and cajoles his friend, "Come on, dude, jump across."

Bob studies the ravine and the distance. Bob's internal computer, his brain, in a few seconds makes an assessment of his fitness and his ability to jump that far. Our bodies have been doing this type of analysis for years—since the first caveman decided what he could climb up or down without getting hurt. Bob's brain reports back to him that his legs can't jump that far.

"Can't do it," he tells Dave and climbs down into the ravine and up the other side.

Our bodies know what's going on. Our bodies make an assessment of what we are able or not able to comfortably do and they tell us, both for jumping across ravines and for far simpler everyday things. They tell us if we listen. They tell us with that little voice in our heads that says:

Don't do that.

You better not do that, you might fall.

Don't put your weight on that side.

You can't do that anymore.

Your knees will give out.

Try to do it another way.

Wait for the elevator.

Not for you.

Let someone else pick it up.

If you do that, it's going to hurt.

These messages are protective devices, but they can also serve as an early warning system of changes in our physical functioning if we stop and listen to them. If we say: "Hmm, isn't that interesting. I used to be able to easily do that and now I can't or don't want to. I wonder why that is."

Pain

If that little voice in our head is the early warning system of changes in our musculoskeletal functioning, then pain is an alarm actually going off. If we persist or are forced to persist in doing something we can no longer comfortably do, the result is pain.

Pain occurs when our alignment is off, when things are rubbing and scraping where they shouldn't, or compensating muscles are getting so fed up with compensating that our bodies let us know loud and clear. Like an unruly child they shout, "I didn't like that!" or "I ain't going to do this anymore, and I'm going to keep telling you until you do something about it."

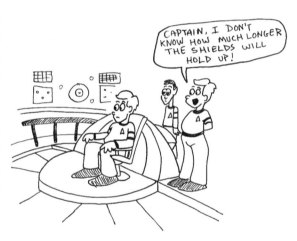

Pain. In any way, shape, or form, whether a dull intermittent ache or a constant roar—pain is a warning sign. Things have progressed to a point where pressure is exceeding the body's tolerances. Red alert!

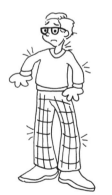

Pain is a warning sign but often we don't listen.

The body reacts. It swells up. It gets inflamed. It develops bursitis and tendonitis. It develops joint pain.

Pain, that's the body's big gun. That's its big attention getter. But too often we still don't listen or snub it out with pain medications.

Does all muscle or joint pain mean a posture problem? Of course not. But as I've said before, lots of muscle and joint pain does. And even if you do have an underlying medical disorder, muscle weakness, stiffness, and malalignment can *contribute* to making it worse.

Am I against pain medications? Of course not. But I am against their continual use to cover up problems that could be treated with postural alignment.

Falling Down And Breaking

If we still don't listen to the pain message—well, our bodies have no choice. They simply stop or they fall down and break. The pain grows so intense, the contracted muscles get so tight, the inflammation goes unchecked for so long that things have to stop. And they do. We can no longer use our elbow or wrist. Our back hurts so much it keeps us out of work. We stop playing tennis. We stop walking. Something pops, snaps, ruptures, or fractures. Something's got to give. As you know by now this often seems to occur out of the blue, but it is really the end result of a progression of events.

When What Feels Normal Isn't

Remember when in the first chapter I said that just because our posture may look the same as many other people's, that doesn't make it normal?

Well, a similar thing happens when we move.

> No matter how aberrant our way of moving, of getting-the-job-done, it invariably feels normal for us.

To be accurate, what *feels* normal is simply what we have grown accustomed to. Remember, muscle weakness and malalignment sneak up on us. Our body's alignment changes by incremental degrees over years, and at each point on the spectrum, we adjust and it begins to feel normal to us. Given enough time, our man's way of walking with the splint on and the marble under his foot will begin to feel normal to him.

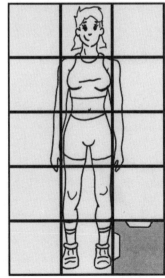

Often we don't recognize or remember what true normal is until we get back to it. That is one of the goals of Posture Alignment.

The Legs Are The First To Go

The legs *are* often the first to go, but they don't need to be. As we grow older, we often feel it in our legs. It's harder to get up when sitting down, it's harder to go up and down stairs, it's harder to balance, and it's harder to bend down and pick things up.

Most of all we feel it in our knees. Our knees are the sentinels of lower extremity malalignment and weakness. They creak, strain, ache, and give way. We blame it on an old football or dance injury.

More often much of this is simply due to weakness in our thigh and leg muscles combined with malalignment. Despite all our walking and sitting and going up and down stairs, our thigh muscles, primarily the quadriceps muscle (the big muscle in front of our thigh), have grown weak. For women in particular, weak quadriceps muscles are also an independent risk factor for osteo-porotic fractures.

If we strengthen the quadriceps muscle along with the other muscles in our legs and correct our alignment, many of our prob-lems will be solved. The big problem with all the quadriceps-strengthening exercises is that they are uncomfortable. They're hard and they hurt.

The Function Menu as well as all of the Lower Extremity exer-cises (both in Chapter 7) address this problem. Try any of the exercises listed for a few days and you will notice a difference.

In the next chapter, we'll take a
look at ideal alignment, and you'll
get the chance to take a closer
look at your own posture . . .

CHAPTER 4

Self-Assessment:How Should the Body Look Anyway?

If you want to cure the soul, cure the body.

– Aristotle

Glad you finally asked. We all have our own idea of what a functional body should look like. What is yours? Six-pack abs? Big muscles? Balance, grace, flexibility? Like a Greek or Roman god or goddess?

All related sciences—anatomy, orthopedics, biomechanics, physical therapy, sports medicine, kineseology— come to the same conclusions on how the body should be aligned for optimal functioning.

Some researchers study the shape of bones, their articulating surfaces, and the alignment and attachments of the muscles. Some pursue lengthy mathematical and computer analyses of vector forces, lines of pull, strength analysis on how and where the body should stand and move for optimal alignment with gravity and performance. Others are more practical: what works, what doesn't work; what causes pain, what doesn't.

They all come to the same conclusions. There is an optimal alignment—an ideal blueprint—where the body works most efficiently and that prevents pain and dysfunction. Variations from that lead to trouble.

> There is an optimal alignment with little variation where our bodies function most efficiently and without pain.

Is it dogmatic to say everyone should look and stand a certain way? Only to the extent that it leads to less disability and a more fully-functional life.

Let's take a quick look at that optimal alignment and then a more detailed look at your own personal alignment.

Overview Of Optimal Alignment

Let's start at the feet and move up: you know, stand on your own two feet, be grounded, and all that.

The feet should point straight ahead or very slightly (up to seven degrees) out to the side. Not flared way out to the side like a duck, or pigeon-toed in. Why? Because the foot is basically a hinge joint designed to operate in the frontal plane. If your feet are significantly turned out and pointing to the sides, for example, when you walk your feet are propelling you laterally while your body is attempting to move forward. This puts a torque or twisting force on your ankles, knees, and hips with every step you take and can cause pain in those areas.

Many people walk with their feet flared out. We may have even been taught to walk that way or have the misconceived notion that it is helpful in sports.

Healthy arches in our feet are a sign of proper alignment and functioning of the muscles that twist and bend the feet and ankles. Collapsed arches can be a sign that we are walking using our hip muscles, throwing our legs forward from the hip with each step, rather than using the muscles in our calves.

The knee joint is another hinge joint that should operate in a plane directly in line with the ankle joint and not be angled inward or outward. The kneecaps are a clue to this alignment; they should be pointing straight ahead. If knees are angled significantly inward or outward, it not only causes more strain on one side of the knee joint and not the other—not a good thing—but also creates a similar twisting force both down to our ankles and up to our hips. Again, one part of our body is trying to go one way and another part is trying to go another way.

Our hips should be level and on the same plane both when seen from the front and when seen from the side. That is, one hip shouldn't be more forward or higher than the other.

Pelvis means basin. If you think of your pelvis as a basin filled with water, it should neither be tipped too far forward nor too far back. When the pelvis is tipped too far forward, the belly often spills over the beltline. When the pelvis is tipped too far back, a person often appears as if they are leading their walk with their pelvis, or as if they are sagging or sitting back in a chair even when they are standing.

The lower back should have a slight arch or concave curve, but not too much and not too little. Like the story of *Goldilocks and the Three Bears*, we don't want too much curve or too little curve; we want it just right.

The chest should be lifted with the shoulders back, not rolled or hunched forward. Think of the upright shoulder positioning in classic Greek and Roman statues. The upper back should have a slight convex curve, but again not be excessively rounded forward.

The head and neck should be in vertical alignment with the rest of the body and not tilted forward, backward, or sideways.

And the body as a whole shouldn't be leaning or appear to be falling forward, backward, or to either side.

Sound pretty complicated? Not really. Here are two pictures: male or female, it doesn't matter. All of our major joints should line up both vertically and horizontally when seen from the front. If you drew a line as in the illustration, the shoulders should be directly above the hip joints, the hip joints should be directly above the knee joints, and the knee joints should be directly above the ankle joints. And no joint should be higher or lower, more forward or backward, or angled when compared to its partner on the other side.

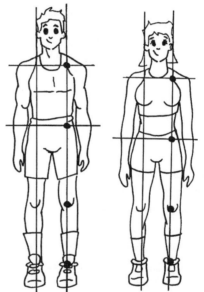

Shoulder joint in line with hip joint

Hip joint directly above knee joint

Knee joint directly above ankle joint

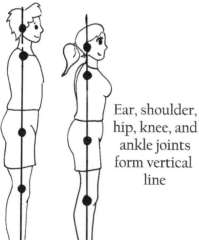

Ear, shoulder, hip, knee, and ankle joints form vertical line

When viewed from the side, a vertical line from the head to the feet should intersect the ankle joint, knee joint, hip joint, shoulder joint, and ear.

Taking A Look At Ourselves

Now is the time you've been waiting for. You get a chance to take a closer look at your own posture. Approach this exercise with a sense of curiosity. Remember, there is no good or bad posture. We are simply seeing different ways our bodies have adjusted to the stresses placed on it. And we can do something about it.

There is a knack to looking at posture or alignment. Don't worry if you can't see everything right away even after doing this exercise. Don't worry if it all doesn't make complete sense. It will make more sense as you go along and soon you too will be become an expert.

How To Do It

The easiest way to see yourself is simply to stand in front of a full-length mirror. It may also be helpful to have a partner, spouse, or friend assist you. They are often able to see and point out things you might miss.

The second way to get a good look at your posture is to take some pictures. A Polaroid or a digital camera works well for this since you can instantly see what's going on. Another major advantage to taking pictures is that you'll have something to compare yourself with and can document your change.

For whatever method you use.

• Ideally wear a bathing suit. Guys don't need a shirt. You want something that reveals your posture so that it isn't hidden underneath folds of clothes. Gym shorts and a leotard also work fine for women.

• Stand in your normal relaxed manner with your feet hip-width apart. No trying to buff your posture for the mirror or camera!

If you are taking pictures:

• Find a wall with a nondescript background.

• Hang a white string with a weight on the end (a plumb line) from the ceiling. This will be our vertical gravity line. A thumbtack works fine to temporarily hold it to the ceiling.

• Take four pictures: one from the front, one from behind, and one from each side.

• Make sure the camera is level with your body and close enough so that your entire body—head to toes—fills the picture.

• For the front shot, stand so that the weight on the string falls directly between your feet. Don't worry about whether it lines up anywhere else. Let your hands relax gently at your sides. Line the string up the same way for the shot from behind.

• For the two pictures from the side, you will want the weight on the string to line up with the bony prominence on the side of your ankle.

Okay, assuming you are standing in front of a mirror or have your pictures ready, let's get started. It's helpful to write down what you see. Don't worry about missing things or messing up. You can always go back and check again. Again, it is the rare person who likes everything they see. We're all out of alignment. From this point on, however, it can only get better.

Let's start by looking at ourselves from the front. Some of the posture disparities in the illustrations which follow are purposely exaggerated. Your posture disparities need be as dramatic (although they may be) for the same principles to apply and for you to benefit by correcting them.

The head should be midline. It shouldn't be leaned or tilted to one side or the other. If it's chronically tilted, some muscles are working overtime.

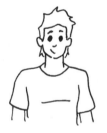

Head
midline

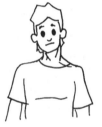

Head always
tilted to
one side

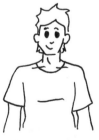

Shoulders
level

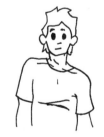

Shoulders <u>not</u>
level - one higher
than the other

The shoulders should be on the same plane when seen from the front. One shouldn't be higher or lower or more forward than the other. Look closely. This is very common and can be subtle. We tend to favor carrying things only on one side—our purses, backpacks, packages, and kids. This can contribute to muscular imbalance and often to shoulder, neck, or upper back pain.

If one shoulder is higher or more forward than the other, do the exercises in the "Asymmetry of Shoulders and Hips—One Shoulder or Hip Higher or More Forward Than the Other" menu in Chapter 7. This takes precedence over any other posture disparity.

Shoulders shouldn't be rolled forward, that is, the front of the shoulders should not be rounded toward you and down. Think of a classic Greek statue again; the shoulders are held up and back. One clue to identifying rounded shoulders is to look at your hands when viewing yourself from the front. Ideally you should see just the sides of your hands from the front, that is, the thumb and the index finger. If you can see part or all of the back of the hand, that often means your shoulders are rolled forward out of position. If you can see the back of one hand and not the other, that means one side is rolled forward or rotated forward more than the other. Rolled forward shoulders are probably one of the most common posture problems you see if you look around. It need not be as dramatic as in the illustration.

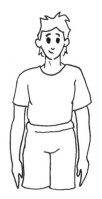

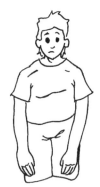

Healthy shoulders not rolled forward

Shoulders rolled forward - can see back of hands from the front

If your shoulders are rolled forward, the "Rounded Shoulders and Upper Back" menu in Chapter 7 will help remedy that.

Next look at your waistline. Your waistline is a clue to the positioning of your pelvis. Is one side higher than the other? This often goes along with one shoulder—either one—being higher than the other (remember the flexible box example in Chapter 2). One side of the pelvis may also appear more forward than the other. You will be able to double-check this from the side view. If your pelvis is not level, you may feel slightly unbalanced when you walk, or may favor using one side over the other when doing activities. Again, it need not be a dramatic as the illustration.

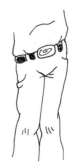

Tilted pelvis as revealed by beltline

> If one side of your pelvis appears more forward or higher than the other, do the exercises in the "Asymmetry of Shoulders and Hips—One Shoulder or Hip Higher or More Forward Than the Other" menu in Chapter 7.

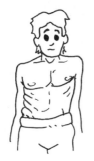

Tilted pelvis - more folds of skin on one side

Also if your midsection is bare, another clue that your pelvis is tilted may be seeing more folds of skin on one side than the other.

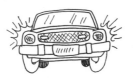 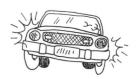

One final test when looking at hip and pelvic positioning from the front is to place a finger on each hip point, the bony prominences in the front of your pelvis. They should be level and both pointing straight ahead like headlights on a car. One shouldn't be angled down or out to the side.

> Do the "Asymmetry of Shoulders and Hips" menu in Chapter 7.

Your knee caps should point straight ahead. If one or both kneecaps point to the side, it means your thigh bones are rotated slightly outward in the hip sockets. If one or both point inward, it means your thigh bones are rotated slightly inward. Either of these may contribute to hip, knee, or ankle pain.

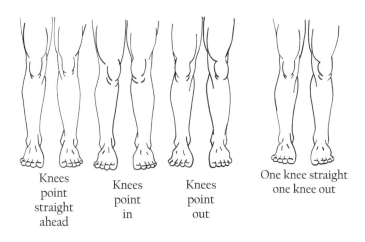

Knees point straight ahead

Knees point in

Knees point out

One knee straight one knee out

> ## The "Knee/Ankle/Foot" menu in Chapter 7 can help with knee malalignment or complaints.

Your ankles should be midline, that is, not rolled in (pronated) or rolled out (supinated). If one or both of your feet are rolled in, you feel the weight on the inside edges of your feet when you walk. If one or both are rolled out, you feel your weight predominately on the outer edges of your feet when you walk. Any disparity here can contribute to foot and ankle problems. Ideally, when you are standing, your weight should be felt equally on both feet. And on each individual foot, your weight should be felt equally front to back and side to side.

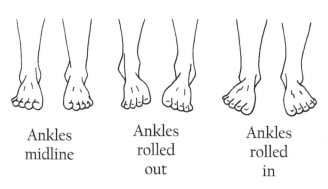

Ankles midline

Ankles rolled out

Ankles rolled in

> ## Consider the "Knee/Ankle/Foot" menu in Chapter 7.

And finally the feet. Your feet should point straight ahead or *very slightly* outward, and not be pointing out to the sides or inward. And the right foot should be the same as the left.

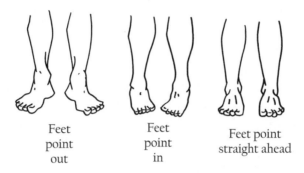

Feet point out

Feet point in

Feet point straight ahead

One quick way to get some clues about your alignment is to sit down and then stand up suddenly. Without adjusting anything, notice your foot position. Is one foot in front of the other? How are your feet pointing? Is your weight more on one side than the other?

> ### For foot problems, consider the "Knee/Ankle/Foot" menu in Chapter 7.

Looking at yourself from behind is mainly useful in confirming some of the things you've noted in the front view. This is where you need to take pictures or have a friend help. One clue for determining whether your ankles are rolled inward or outward is to look at your Achilles tendon, that big tendon behind your heel. Ideally, it should be close to vertical. If it forms an angle just above your heel, that can be a sign that your ankles are rolled.

On the back view also look again for angulation of the shoulders and hips from the horizontal. Sometimes it is easier to see this problem from behind.

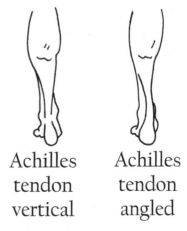

Achilles tendon vertical

Achilles tendon angled

Now let's look at the side view. Ideally, take pictures or have a friend help for this one too, since you will have to alter your posture to turn to the side to look.

Remember, in our ideal man or woman a plumb line or weighted string from the ceiling should intersect the following points from the side: ankles, knees, hips, shoulders, and ears.

The body should be vertical. That is, the whole body should neither be leaning forward of the string nor behind it. Look closely. More often we have some parts that line up with the string and other parts that fall forward or lag behind the string.

The head should be upright, not jutted forward of the vertical line of the body. If the head is too far forward, it can cause strain and pain in the muscles behind the neck and in the shoulders.

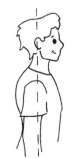

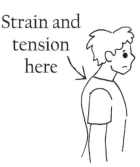

Strain and tension here

Head midline and upright

Head and neck jutted forward

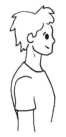

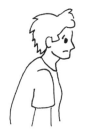

Shoulders positioned correctly

Rolled forward shoulders and rounded upper back

It is often much easier to see rolled-forward shoulders on the side view. If you're wearing a T-shirt with a seam running down the top of your shoulder, that seam should run directly down the center of your shoulder until it hits the sleeve. A rounded or hunched upper back often goes along with rolled shoulders giving the body a carrying-the-weight-of-the-world appearance.

The "Rounded Shoulders and Upper Back" menu in Chapter 7 will help remedy a forward head, rounded shoulders, or hunched upper back.

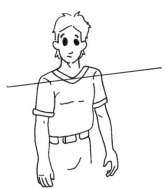

Both shoulders should be on the same plane as the head and torso. Just as one shoulder shouldn't be higher than the other, one shoulder shouldn't be more forward than the other. One clue to identifying this problem is seeing more of the back in one side view than in the other.

One shoulder
more forward
and lower than
the other

> If one shoulder is higher or more forward than the other, do the exercises in the "Asymmetry of Shoulders and Hips—One Shoulder or Hip Higher or More Forward Than the Other" menu in Chapter 7. This takes precedence over any other disparity.

Next let's look at the pelvis from the side. There are three possibilities: your pelvis is neutral, that is, horizontal and positioned correctly; your pelvis is tilted too far forward; or your pelvis is tilted too far backward. Again, your beltline offers a valuable clue. Ideally, the belt on your clothing should be close to horizontal.

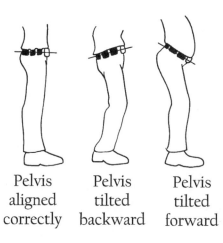

Pelvis   Pelvis   Pelvis
aligned   tilted   tilted
correctly   backward   forward

If your pelvis is tilted too far forward, you will generally have an exaggerated curve (too much curve) in your lower back. Often the person with a forward-tilted pelvis has trouble putting their low back completely flat when lying down on the floor or when standing backward up against a wall.

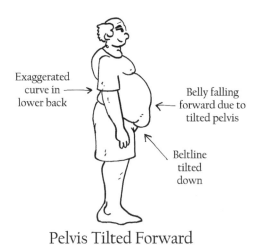

Exaggerated curve in → lower back

Belly falling ← forward due to tilted pelvis

Beltline tilted down

Pelvis Tilted Forward

Another clue to a pelvis tilted too far forward is a gut hanging over your beltline. This may not be just from over-eating. When a pelvis is tilted forward, the abdominal wall isn't strong enough nor is it designed to keep everything from spilling forward.

A pelvis that is tilted forward means the muscles that connect the legs to the upper body in our groins are too tight. Like powerful rubberbands they continually jackknife the torso and legs together.

> ### The "Pelvis Tilted Forward" menu in Chapter 7 will help remedy this.

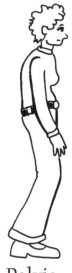

Pelvis tilted backward

If your pelvis is tilted backward, you have the opposite problem. You won't have enough curve in your lower back. Your back will be flat when you lie on the floor. A person with a backward-tilted pelvis looks as if they are sitting or sagging backward. It appears as if their muscles are too weak to hold the body up and their upper body collapses and sags backward and down into itself.

Clues for the backward-tilting pelvis also include loss of prominence of gluteal tissue, that is, poor definition of the buttocks. Older people often tend to wear their pants or slacks higher and higher on their waists because of the increasingly backward tilt of their pelvis. Loss of the curve in the lower back and the corresponding loss of gluteal prominence leads to their pants wanting to continually slide down. With a backward-tilting pelvis, a belt around the waist often appears higher in the front than in the back.

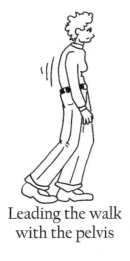

With the backward tilt, the pelvis is sometimes (not always) pushed forward, that is, displaced anteriorly as if the person is leading their walk with their pelvis.

Leading the walk
with the pelvis

> The "Pelvis Tilted Backward" menu in
> Chapter 7 will help remedy this.

The pelvis is like a rocker. If it is rocked too far forward, the center of gravity is displaced too far forward and the positioning of everything above and below it is altered. If it is tilted too far back, the center of gravity is too far back. (See ITPS: "It's the Pelvis, Silly" at the end of this chapter)

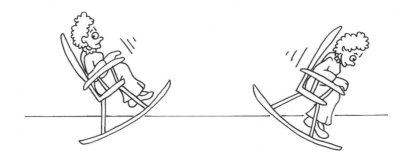

Our pelvis needs to be able to readily tilt both forward and backward, for example, when we walk. But we don't want it locked in a too-far-forward or a too-far-backward position on a chronic basis. If you want to get the feeling of a pelvis tilted too far forward, grab your pelvic bones from the side, fingers forward and thumbs behind. Now, while keeping the rest of your body steady, rock just your pelvic bone forward accentuating the arch in your back. That is a pelvis tilted too far forward.

For a backward-tilted pelvis, tilt your hands and your pelvic bone backward, jutting your whole pelvis forward. That is an exaggerated backward tilt.

Seen from the side, our knees shouldn't be overly flexed (bent), or overly straight (hyperextended). We want them right in the middle.

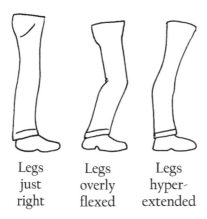

Legs just right   Legs overly flexed   Legs hyper-extended

For knee malalignment, consider the "Knee/Ankle/Foot" menu in Chapter 7.

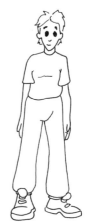

And finally, the feet again. One foot shouldn't be forward of the other. This most often means that farther up the line at the hip, one hip is higher or more forward than the other.

Standing with one foot always forward of the other

Do the exercises in the "Asymmetry of Shoulders and Hips" menu in Chapter 7.

Discouraged or confused? Not to worry. Again, don't feel you have to see everything right now, or that you might be missing something? If you pick up one or two things or just start to get a feel for this, that's fine for now.

Maybe you feel you may have too many areas off? "Jeez, I see everything he's talking about. I'm supposed to do all the menus!" Don't worry. It will all be explained as we go along.

> Feel you have too many areas off? Trust me—
> wherever you are is fine. From here on out
> things will only get better.

For now, the main things you want to decide while looking at yourself are whether you have asymmetry of your shoulders and hips (one shoulder or hip higher or more forward than the other—it doesn't matter which one) and whether your pelvis is level or tilted forward or backward.

To repeat, asymmetry of shoulder and hips reveals itself by either one shoulder or hip being higher or lower than the other on the front or back views, or more forward or backward than the other on the side views. Remember the flexible box example in Chapter 2—if there is a twist in your shoulders, there is invariably some twist in your pelvis, although it may subtle and harder to see. If there is a twist in your pelvis, there has to be some twist in your shoulders too.

The second thing you want to look for is whether your pelvis is level, tilted forward, or tilted backward. Look at other people. Try to pick out which ones have a forward-tilted pelvis, which ones have a backward tilt, and which ones are neutral. On some people it is dramatic and easy to see, on others it is more subtle. Remember lots of arch in the low back and a tilted-forward beltline are two clues for the forward-tilted pelvis.

The backward-tilted pelvis often goes along with rounded shoulders and upper back. It is very common, particularly among men and women who are sedentary and sit for long periods of time.

> No matter what you see you can improve,
> and it will make a difference in your life.

Perhaps, while you were doing this self-examination, you tried to correct some of the areas that looked off. But you quickly fell back into malalignment. We may hold good posture for a few seconds or minutes even but we soon collapse back down.

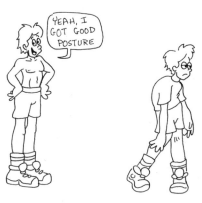

Why is this? Again, it's because certain muscles aren't strong enough to hold us where we should be. Those muscles need to be strengthened. And certain areas are too tight. Like bowstrings they pull us back out of alignment. Those areas need to be loosened up and stretched.

How Disparities In Posture Feel

Alterations in our posture often have symptoms that go along with them. Here are a few.

Head forward: Strain or tension in the back of your neck or upper back; headaches.

Shoulders rolled forward or shoulders not level: Tension and tightness in the shoulders and upper back; symptoms in the elbows, wrists, and hands often including abnormal sensations, tingling, and pain.

Hunched upper back: Pain and tension in the upper back muscles.

One shoulder higher or more forward than the other: Any of the above symptoms as well as tension or tightness in one flank region.

Hips rotated: Feeling more weight on one foot more than the other, or more weight on the front of side of one foot than the other. You will often tend to favor one leg over the other, using it to carry most of your weight or do most of the work. Another clue for this is the way you walk; your cadence or the sound of your walk may not be equal or sound symmetrical. One leg may be swinging faster than the other. If your hips aren't level, it can lead to pain in your hips, knees, ankles, or feet.

Whole body forward or backward of the plumb line: Feeling as if you are constantly falling forward or backward and have to hold yourself up, producing tension or strain in upper or lower back and flank muscles.

Pelvis tilted too far forward: Pain, strain, and tension in the low back.

Pelvis tilted too far backward: Trouble getting up from a sitting position. Lower back pain.

Knees turned out or in: One knee or ankle may hurt or be prone to injury.

Everted feet: One or both feet may hurt or be prone to injury.

Virtually any and all aches or pains may be brought on by faulty alignment.

ITPS: "It's The Pelvis, Silly"

It's always the pelvic bone that controls our alignment destiny in the world of functional alignment. It's always the pelvis.

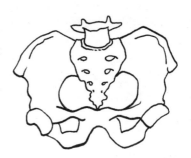

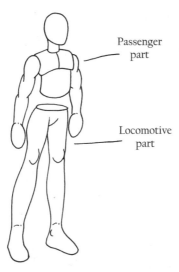

Passenger part

Locomotive part

The pelvis has been described as a platform in the center of the body. The top part of our body is a passenger who rides on top of this platform. The bottom of our body is the locomotive part that moves us forward. Big muscles from above and below intersect at the platform with our body's center of gravity residing just above the pelvis.

Anatomically, in an aligned pelvis, a line connecting the tip of the tailbone (coccyx) and the point where the pubic bones meet in the front (pubic symphysis) should be horizontal. And the hip points (anterior superior iliac spines) should form a vertical line with the pubic symphysis.

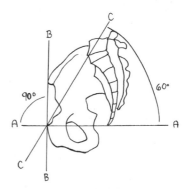

Any alteration in the alignment of this platform causes a cascade of potentially detrimental effects both above and below the pelvis.

Pelvis leaned too far forward . . . the whole structure above and below gets out of line and starts toppling forward. The body has to compensate to remain upright.

Pelvis tilted too far back . . . same thing. The body sags backward and the whole structure wants to topple backward and the shoulders and head roll forward to compensate.

Pelvis cocked to one side (one hip higher or more forward than the other) . . . a twisting force is applied all the way up to our shoulders and neck and along our backs and down through our legs. Everything above and below by definition is thrown out of line and feels the strain from this malalignment.

This is why as you correct your pelvic alignment, other alterations in your posture will automatically begin to correct themselves. This is also why so many of the Posture Alignment exercises focus on the pelvis.

But let's move on. There is hope. We can change
and correct all these things . . . but first
we have to see why we can't just randomly
exercise and expect to fix things, and why
the healthcare system can't be our ultimate savior.

CHAPTER **5**

Why There's More To It Than Just Do It

*The neglect of physical exercise is held,
by leading medical authorities to be producing
the gravest results in this country.*

— *Health Lift* Brochure, 1875

So why not just get out there and jog, lift weights, or take some exercise class at your local health club?

Because . . . random exercise won't correct postural malalignment. Exercise may help your heart and lungs, make some muscles stronger, and give you a dose of much-needed motion, but if your alignment is off, it won't make it right. And, despite what I said about the need to move, it might even make things worse.

> Random exercise won't correct postural malalignment.
> It takes focused exercise to correct our posture.
> And as long as you are out of alignment,
> you remain a candidate for the downward spiral.

Buffing Your Dysfunctions

Yes, it's true. You could exercise for days and weeks and months and years and actually put yourself farther down the road to dysfunction. When our bodies are out of alignment, if we aren't careful, all our actions tend to reinforce and perpetuate our dysfunctions.

For example, if your upper back is hunched over to begin with, and you ride an exercise bike, you will tend to do it in a hunched-over position. This reinforces the positioning of the muscles that keep you hunched over. If you are out of alignment, weight lifting can strengthen the muscles that keep you that way.

Exercising in
hunched forward position
may perpetuate
rounded upper back

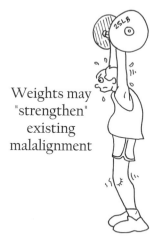

Weights may
"strengthen"
existing
malalignment

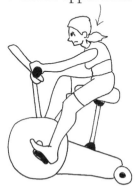

Weight machines and free weights in particular should have warning signs on them. Use at your own risk. These are powerful tools.

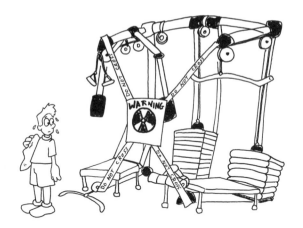

In any physical activity, we naturally favor using our strong muscles—getting the job done with the muscles that are already strong—and avoid using our weak muscles. Stiffness and inflexibility often prevent us from accessing and using the muscles we need to use. The rich get richer and the poor get poorer.

> Strong muscles get stronger and weak muscles
> get weaker. Stiff areas remain stiff. Abnormalities in
> our posture remain or become more pronounced.

Just as our personality often becomes hardened and more fixed as we grow older, so does our posture. Whatever small abnormalities we may have in our postural alignment become more exaggerated. A cocked head becomes more cocked. Rolled-forward shoulders become more rolled forward. A pelvis that tilts backward tilts backward even more. Any cracks in our structure become deeper and more pronounced as we grow older.

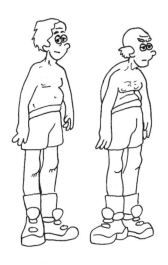

> With random exercise you risk making your
> strong parts stronger and your weak parts weaker,
> hence perpetuating any malalignment in your posture.

All the gyrating and twisting you see at the average health club are attempts to enlist the already strong muscles to do the job—another version of the compensation we talked about before.

The same thing can happen in exercise classes. In an attempt to keep up with the teacher or the music we tend to do whatever is necessary to get the job done, often not using the muscles we should. We move within our set range-of-motion boxes, albeit faster and perhaps to music, but still within our own boxes.

And even if you do all of your exercises with meticulously correct alignment—feet pointing straight ahead, etc.—although that would help, it won't get you back into alignment. Before weak muscles can be strengthened and properly aligned, space must be created. And that means stretching and opening things up. Not by a few brief attempts to reach down and touch your toes—but with deeper, more controlled forms of stretching to open up the tight areas.

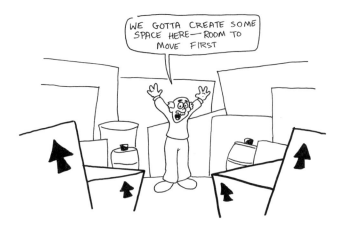

Then, in that new space, the proper muscles can be strengthened and aligned. That is why Posture Alignment combines exercises that first stretch us followed by exercises that strengthen and align.

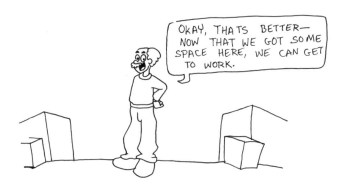

Our Legs Can't Keep Up With Our Lungs

Another thing often happens when you decide to climb onto that exercise bike or start jogging again. Your cardiovascular system (your heart and lungs) often adapts faster than the rest of your body does.

Over several days or weeks, your heart and lungs adapt but unfortunately you are still left with the tilted pelvis or rounded back. Weak and mal-aligned muscle groups are forced to compensate as best they can. We do things such as swinging one leg around in a wide arc to carry most of our weight or having one side do most of the work. And although our endurance and strength may increase, if we are really honest with ourselves, this is why it still doesn't feel quite right and is often no fun.

> When a demand is placed on us, we are
> immediately forced to compensate.

Let me interject here that I have the utmost respect for anyone who exercises, anyone who does anything to maintain his or her health. I know the time and effort involved. Anyone who makes any effort to improve or maintain their health is a hero in my mind.

Posture Alignment isn't opposed to exercise and I don't mean to convey a snob-bish or elitist attitude with regard to posture or correct alignment. Rather, by align-ing ourselves *first*, we bring more efficiency and results to our chosen exercise program. By aligning ourselves, we are able to do more and enjoy it more.

> Correct your postural alignment and all
> exercises and sports will become a million
> times easier and more fun!

We Often Avoid What We Really Need

It's human nature. We avoid the exercises and activities that are "hard" for us—the ones where we can't cheat. Or we do them so rarely that they don't have a chance to have a lasting effect on our alignment.

> If an exercise is "hard" for us, it usually
> means it requires us to use muscles that we
> haven't been using, and that is often
> the exercise we need to do.

And a corollary to this is . . .

> The exercises we can't do or don't
> want to do reveal our dysfunctions.

If a certain movement is difficult for you, it's a sign that you are deficient in the strength, flexibility, or alignment needed for that movement. It should make you curious and perhaps want to correct that deficiency.

Focus On Appearance

One of the greatest dangers of blindly "buying into" the fitness industry advertising is often its sole focus on appearance. Products are sold based on how they might make us look. A certain appearance—big biceps, a sculpted body, six-pack abs, buns of steel—is often equated with fitness or health. If I could get my body to look this way, then I'd be fit, right?

> An attractive appearance does not necessarily
> equate with functional fitness.

Even the phrase "physical fitness" calls to mind its minions—air-brushed twenty-something year olds with abs and butts of steel hoisting shiny weights on beaches or pumping away on the exercise machines du jour. The rippled, muscular guy is seen as healthy; the buff magazine-cover woman with a thin sheen of perspiration is seen as fit.

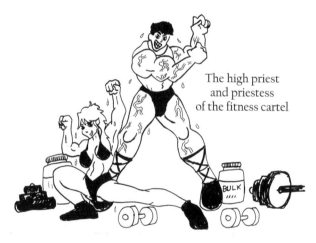

The high priest
and priestess
of the fitness cartel

While an inherently functional, attractive, and aligned body can be the result of Posture Alignment, that is not our sole goal. Our goal includes maximizing our function and minimizing pain and disability.

> Our goal, along with improving our appearance,
> is to maximize our musculoskeletal function allowing
> us to comfortably do a wide variety of activities for
> as long as possible while minimizing and
> preventing musculoskeletal disability.

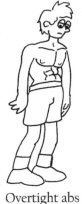

Overtight abs
contributing to
backward pelvic
tilt

To do an exercise to enlarge or shape only a certain part of the body to the exclusion of all other parts, along with being adolescent, can also be absurd and dangerous.

For example, to work on strengthening the abdominal muscles for appearance alone can lead to imbalance. There are other muscle groups, both on the back and on the front of the body, that balance the effects of the abdominal muscles. By over-strengthening and ratcheting the abdominals tighter, we risk distorting our alignment.

> Focusing on appearance to the exclusion of alignment or function is absurd. It can lead to further malalignment and dysfunction.

Why Do All Exercise Programs Seem To Work—Sometimes

All exercise programs seem to work for some people some of the time. For any given exercise regime there are some people who swear by it while others who, despite persistent effort, make little real progress.

People who succeed in a given exercise program more often arrive with the attributes (strength and flexibility) required for that activity. There is often a self-selection process present in exercise classes and sports. Those who can do the activity do it and persist in it, while those who can't, drop out. Dance students tend to flock to yoga and thrive since they already have much of the core strength and flexibility required. Those who don't have these attributes often drop out after a few sessions.

> People tend to persist in exercise programs in which they already have at least some of the muscular strength, flexibility, and coordination required.

In many exercise programs, the exercises that would address a person's individual dysfunctions are too diffuse. It may be possible to get back into alignment but it will take a very long time—more time and dedication than most people are able to give.

The real test of any exercise program should be: How many average people it can take off the street and bring them back to function in the shortest amount of time?

And while various exercises and classes come in and go out of vogue, the basic principles of alignment do not, cannot, and will not change. And only to the extent that a given exercise program addresses those principles will it be useful long term.

> The Posture Alignment principles are universal.
> They work. They can't not work.

The Fitness Cartel

Finally, remember that the fitness industry is a business. Their goal is to make money. In general, they will sell us anything related to health or fitness that they can make money on.

Any exercise program or class is a tool. Pick and choose the tools that will be most useful for you keeping in mind the principles of postural alignment. Use the tools with awareness. Use the tools in a manner which contributes to and doesn't detract from postural alignment.

> Choose carefully your health and fitness tools.
> Use them in a manner which contributes
> to maintaining proper alignment.

Now let's take a look at why modern medicine can never really cure us—at least our muscles and bones—without our doing something for ourselves.

Modern Medicine

Modern healthcare is indeed miraculous. Breakthroughs in science combined with increasing technical skills and equipment enamor us each day with what is possible. And it seems that it should be increasingly easy for *them* to fix us when we hurt or break down.

We want to be able to take our bodies in to the shop, just like our cars when they break down, and have someone fix them as quickly as possible and get us back out there.

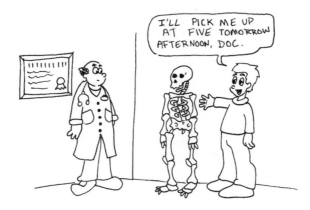

But I don't suspect you'd be reading this book or have gotten this far if you thought that's all there was to it. Maybe you've had your own experience. Maybe you've gone through your own progression of doctors or healthcare providers and felt that no one ever really got to the root of the problem. The solutions were palliative at best.

Here are some key points to remember about the healthcare system:

• If we aren't careful, medicine often dissociates ourselves . . . from ourselves. If we aren't careful, we may be led to believe that we somehow don't have anything to do with what's going on, nor can we have any real effect on it.

> If we aren't careful, the health care system usurps a great deal of our power and authority over ourselves.

When it comes to our musculoskeletal health, these views can be disastrous.

> We have a considerable stake in what's going on with our muscles and bones, and we can control and correct a great number of our muscle and joint problems ourselves.

• Simple solutions are the best. It makes sense to correct things in the least invasive way possible. If we can correct a great deal of our musculoskeletal complaints by staying flexible, strong, and in alignment, why not do that?

Instead, many people choose the path of decreased activity (the downward spiral), increased use of pain medicines (with their adverse effects), and orthopedic surgery.

No question—orthopedists are wizards with muscle, bone, ligaments, and tendons. They can shave off bone, use tendons for ligaments, and replace parts with plastic and titanium. They can reconstruct and even replace entire joints. But you don't want to have them do all those things unless you have to. Additional limitations brought on by surgery can sometimes only compound problems.

> The simplest, least invasive solutions
> are most often the best.

• It is always wisest to fix problems at the earliest stage possible using the simplest means possible, while preserving as much of the original function as possible. If we can correct our problems by exercising and aligning ourselves, that is always the wisest solution.

> Before buying into the mindset that something
> is permanently and irrevocably wrong with
> your knees, back, or shoulders, seriously consider
> the possibility that you need to strengthen
> and align those parts of your body first.

• Often the underlying causes that precipitated a problem are never addressed (muscle weakness, loss of flexibility, loss of correct postural alignment).

> If you never address the true underlying problem,
> you can never solve a problem for the long term.

Much of our disability that seemingly occurs out of the blue is an outgrowth of weakness and faults in our alignment. There is often a long progression when we don't feel anything unusual but where things are getting out of line. There are many points along the way where we can do something.

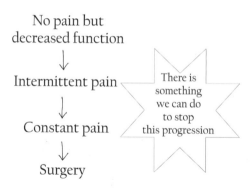

No pain but
decreased function

↓

Intermittent pain

↓

Constant pain

↓

Surgery

There is
something
we can do
to stop
this progression

Muscle weakness and postural malalignment are, if not the cause, chief contributing factors to many of our musculoskeletal aches and pains and much of our subsequent dysfunction.

Hunched, rounded upper backs can lead to pain and tension in our necks and shoulders. Rounded shoulders and decreased range of motion in our shoulders contribute to rotator cuff tears and carpal tunnel syndrome. A pelvis that is tilted too far forward or backward can contribute to lower back and hip pain. A weak, mal-aligned back is one that is prone to injury. Legs that are mal-aligned can cause knee, ankle, and foot pain or injury. Weak muscles and loss of balance all contribute to falling. The list goes on and on.

> Modern healthcare is miraculous. But it can't give you back or maintain your musculoskeletal health. You have to do that yourself.

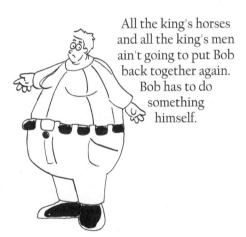

All the king's horses and all the king's men ain't going to put Bob back together again. Bob has to do something himself.

• Be careful! Pain medicines often cover up a problem by forcing it off to the side until it worsens enough to compel us to pay attention. Remember, pain is a warning signal that something is off, something is wrong. I am no hero. There is no question that pain medications are useful during any acute injury, and certainly there are many people with chronic muscle and joint diseases for whom pain medications are lifesavers. But . . . for most of us, if you are using pain medications on a regular basis for a musculoskeletal problem, be wary. You may simply be covering something up that will get worse.

> Pain is a warning from the body. Pain pills cover this up and are a temporary fix while under the surface things can be getting worse.

Just as it would be foolish to take pain medications to cover up a problem with our heart or intestines, it is the same with our musculoskeletal system.

• Alternative medicine is often no different. While useful adjuncts, no amount of manipulation, massage therapy, acupuncture, or herbal remedies will make weak muscles strong, stiff muscles flexible, and align your posture. We often don't want to hear it, but regardless of what is done to you, if you don't strengthen a weak muscle, it simply won't hold you up properly. That's all there is to it.

> Insofar as alternative medicine doesn't address our alignment and correct our muscular weaknesses and imbalances, it can't provide a long-term solution.

• Finally, to be fair and balance things out, let's face it, we—as patients—often contribute to all of the above. Frequently we aren't willing to do what it takes— particularly if it involves consistent effort or time on our part. We demand and accept the quick fix, the pain pills, and the surgery even if they aren't in our own best long term interest. But again, I doubt if you would have gotten this far in this book if you were willing to settle for that.

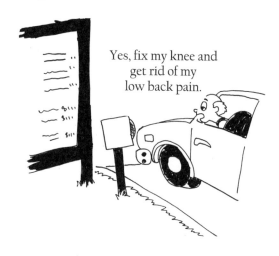

At last! Chapter 6 offers a solution.

There is an answer.

The Solution

If anything is sacred, the human body is sacred.

— Walt Whitman

The Good News—Everything We Need Is Still There

We haven't lost any muscles or bones. Nothing has fallen away or disappeared. Everything is still attached where it is supposed to be.

And we haven't worn down our bodies. Despite what we would like to believe, most of us haven't physically worked so hard our entire lives that some parts have truly worn out. The great majority of us have experienced no devastating musculoskeletal illness or trauma.

Everything is still there, ready to go. It simply hasn't been fully used in a while. Like state-of-the-art spaceships parked in dry dock, everything is ready to go given half a chance.

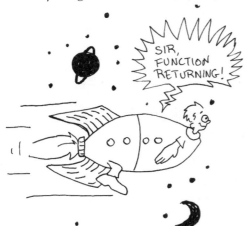

Given a little stimulation the control panel will light up. A little more stimulation and engineering will report, "Sir, we have power."

"Life support systems working and fully functional," an ensign on another deck reports.

Fire up the booster rockets. We become functional again.

The real miracle of the human body is its ability to recover, to regain lost functions. We are truly blessed that although functions may seem lost, they are not lost forever. Rather, they are placed in a state of quiescence that may extend to forever if we don't do anything about it.

> There is nothing more encouraging than
> the body's ability to recover and regain
> its functions when given half a chance.

The Body Wants To Go Home

The second encouraging fact is that the body is on our side. It wants to go home, Dorothy. It is not as if there are umpteen possible ways for the body to function and do things and we have to somehow find the one that works. The body knows. There is a "home" that it craves to return to.

> Our bodies want to go home.

Despite any number of glitches, despite any amount of abuse or disregard, we have built-in homing devices for optimal function. All these wanderings outside have been trying on our bodies too. Proper body alignment and coordinated movement is the most useful, efficient, and economical use of energy and resources; our bodies want to go back home as much as we do.

Given half a chance—like salmon finding the same stream—our bodies will find their way back to functional alignment.

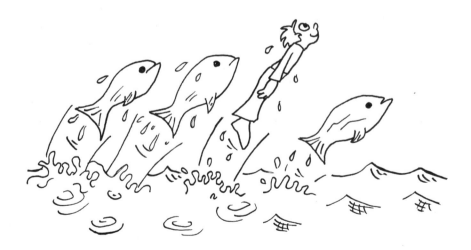

How The Body Gets Back Into Alignment

Slowly. Gradually. By degrees.

It's taken you a while to get yourself into the shape you are in—years, decades, all your life. And it takes a while to return to normal.

The return to proper alignment is an incremental process. One part often can't correct until another part corrects first. If one shoulder is higher than another, our shoulders don't suddenly pop back into correct position. Rather, our hips have to give up a little bit of their tightness, which then allows our shoulders to correct slightly. This allows our hips to realign even more. And on it goes, small incremental change in one area allowing change in other areas.

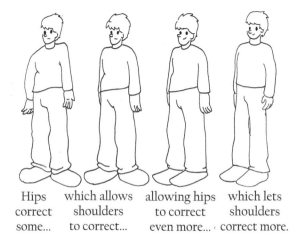

| Hips correct some... | which allows shoulders to correct... | allowing hips to correct even more... | which lets shoulders correct more. |

Remember in the flexible box model how if one part bends, the rest of the structure has to bend somewhere else. To reverse the process, one part often can't release or let go until another part releases and lets go.

Another useful analogy is to think of a tumbler lock on a big bank vault door. For the lock to open all the tumblers inside have to line up. It's often the same with our bodies. The hips can't release until the shoulders move back a little and the quads are stretched out some. Then, ca-chunk, your hip can move back some more.

So how long does it take to re-align your body? It all depends on where you start from and how much you apply yourself. Can everyone achieve perfect posture? No. Some people are too stiff, or too old, or won't do the exercises enough.

But everyone can improve their alignment—usually dramatically—and consequently improve their appearance, and increase their function and enjoyment of activities. And that is what matters.

Remember, if you are in pain due to malalignment, any little change in your posture may be enough to alleviate all or at least some of the pain.

Which leads us to . . .

It Has To Feel Weird

Homeostasis is a fancy word for "where we are at." The first part of the word is home and that's exactly what it is to us. No big changes. Nothing to upset the status quo. And we often hope it will remain that way. Homeostasis can be applied to your present level of strength, flexibility, and alignment.

But just as you have to leave home to grow up, you have to leave your comfort zone to become stronger, more flexible, and more in line.

And just as it feels uncomfortable or different when we leave home or do something new, our body has to feel "different" when we start to make changes in our alignment.

If you do the exercises which follow, you will feel your weight shifting from where it was before. You may feel new sensations or soreness in a muscle you aren't used to using. The way you walk may feel different. These things mean that you are beginning to use muscles or portions of muscles that you may not have used for some time.

These are all signs that we are indeed making changes—that the exercises are doing something. And I suggest that you court these strange feelings because they indicate that something indeed is happening. Paydirt. That's what we want. These feelings are clues that change is occurring. Posture Alignment requires that you go through periods of time when your body is readjusting and it can feel strange.

> To get from here to there you have to go through here.

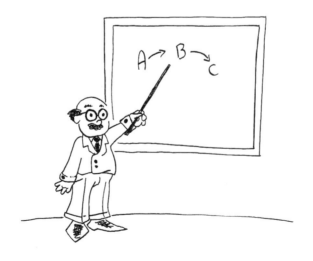

And even though your body does want to get back to its design template, it can become a little confused when you start messing with it. After all it has gotten comfortable where it is.

Take a habit you do every day like brushing your teeth with your right hand and try doing it with your left hand. Suddenly you are uncoordinated and your body doesn't like it.

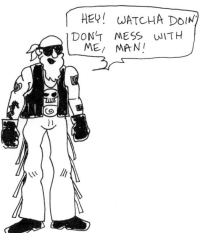

It has to feel weird or different.
That means things are changing.

Or to put it another way, if nothing happens, if it never feels weird or difficult or strange or slightly uncomfortable, that means you aren't changing anything.

If it doesn't feel weird, strange, or different,
it probably means you aren't doing anything.

Pain

If an activity is truly painful, don't do it. That's all there is to it. Hopefully the person who invented the maxim, "No pain, no gain," is long gone after having suffered a most painful demise. After all we certainly have enough pain in our lives without actively courting it in an exercise program.

The problem however is that many of us have become well . . . a little numb to what is really pain. We are often quick to interpret any sensation in our bodies that is different as being pain, or bad, or something wrong. Not everything new we feel in our bodies is bad. An odd feeling is not always pain; it's just different. Sometimes we aren't used to the sensation of our body simply working hard or stretching near its limits.

In particular, it can often be hard to distinguish these two when starting or restarting an exercise program. While I want to caution you particularly at first to err on the side of being too careful, at the same time, please recognize that a certain amount of effort is involved improving your alignment. It has to hurt a little or at least feel a bit uncomfortable at times.

Our muscles become stronger by being overloaded. We become more flexible by over-stretching. Lifting weights well below your threshold or stretching well within your limits won't do anything. You *do* have to push yourself a little to get results.

With regard to stretching, there's a pain when things can go no further, or at least not right now and there is a sensation where things are tight and can be stretched. This is where you come in. Again, carefully, cautiously you need to figure out the difference between those two—for yourself.

If an activity or exercise is painful, go back and reevaluate what you're doing. Perhaps try an easier, milder version of the exercise. If something hurts badly, see your doctor. Use your own best judgment. I trust you to know.

> ## If it is painful, don't do it.

Snap, Crackle, And Pop

You know what I'm talking about here—the way your joints sound—all that creaking, straining, grinding, snapping, popping, and cracking.

Sometimes it sounds like one of those old World War II submarine movies where the submarine is trapped well below its designated depth and the whole hull starts creaking and straining. Any moment we expect rivets to begin popping out and water to start rushing in.

I know the sounds sound scary like something bad is happening. Like we might be making things worse or, indeed, like something might blow. And when we hear those noises our joints make, there is a tendency to want to stop.

But not to worry. Given a little common sense, these are good sounds. The same old rule applies: if it isn't painful, don't worry about it. After all, people pay chiropractors to produce those noises and here we are—getting them for free.

There are lots of explanations for these noises and I guess you could attempt to categorize each and every one of them. Common explanations include the breaking up of small deposits of calcium, slight repositioning of the bone in the joint, tendons and ligaments running over areas of constriction and repositioning themselves, and cavitation effects from the negative pressure of water in joints (now that does sound scary!).

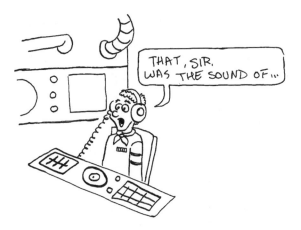

If it doesn't hurt, if there isn't bad pain associated with it, then don't worry about it. These are the signs of things getting back into place and they should be a welcome sound to your ears. And often most of them will go away.

> You will hear noises.

Kinesthetic Sense

When we start doing something to get our bodies back into alignment, particularly if we haven't done anything for a long time, our sense of our bodies, our kinesthetic sense, is often blunted or has gone slightly numb.

Our nerves may be frazzled and weary from pain and we may have partially shut ourselves off from our bodies. We don't know what we feel. It is as if we are wearing three or four winter coats and several pairs of mittens.

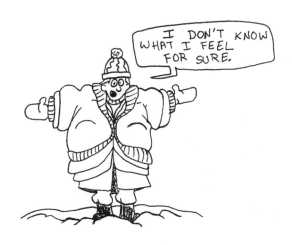

We don't know where our weight is when we stand. We can't see or feel one shoulder or hip being higher or lower than the other. We can't tell what muscles we are using to do what. Our bodies may have even become amorphous globs "down there" somewhere below our heads.

And just because we already exercise doesn't necessarily mean we are immune from this. Many people put their bodies through their paces without being totally conscious of them.

At first, when you do some of the Posture Alignment exercises, your alignment and positioning may only be a gross approximation like an artist's initial rough sketch. But over time, your kinesthetic sense will return. With your return to alignment, you will become more aware of where your weight is and what muscles you are using. Your ability to align yourself for the exercises and throughout the day will improve.

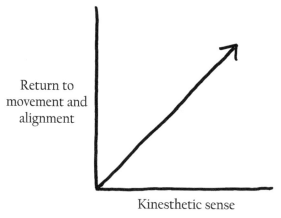

Return to movement and alignment

Kinesthetic sense

> With our return to alignment,
> our kinesthetic sense improves and increases.

It's important to let our bodies figure things out.

When we first try a new movement that we aren't used to, we often feel clumsy and uncoordinated. Our bodies sway this way and that. We put our weight here and then there. We try to use this muscle then that one. We wobble. We fall. This is the body's way of figuring things out. It goes too far in one direction, then too far in the other direction, and eventually over time figures things out.

We knew this as kids but we often forget it as adults. Like a child, give your body and yourself room to experiment, to learn. Don't be too quick to decide that just because you can't do an exercise or activity perfect immediately, you can't do it at all. Don't assume nothing is being gained by the trying process.

> Give your body time and space to figure things out.

Is our internal dialogue riddled with "Oh, you stupid klutz!" "You can't do that," or "I don't have good balance. No one in my family has good balance, you know." Whatever your own favorite negative phrases are put them aside. Give this process room to work.

As I said before, we have evolved over millions of years, and it doesn't make sense that we would come this far with some of us being totally deficient in key abilities.

> Rather than blaming anything you can't do on an inherent deficiency, simply tell yourself that certain muscles are weak, certain areas are tight, and you simply haven't done it enough. When you correct those things, you will be able to do it.

Coordination in great part comes from simply doing an activity. Exercise physiologists use the term muscle memory to describe this. Our muscles figure out the correct sequence of contracting and releasing to do an activity and it becomes easier. Granted, for some this occurs faster than for others. But we all have it. The greatest fallacy is to try an exercise or activity a few times and then give up on it, or blame our failure on some inherent deficiency.

> Give your self the time and space to figure things out.

You Are The Ultimate Expert
With Regard To Your Own Body

Yes, you are the ultimate expert with regard your own body. But you already knew that. I'm not quite ready to say, "Close this book, and trust the Force, Luke." But I do believe that if we listen to ourselves, most of us do know more than we think.

We can feel what exercises are best for us. We can tell when they are working. We know which ones, although slightly uncomfortable, are good for us and getting us back into alignment. We know what is a good type of hurt that means things are stretching, and when we should stop.

That's why, in the exercise section of this book, there are often several alternative exercises. I encourage you to be open to what works best for you.

And this applies while doing any individual exercise as well. Listen and trust that little voice that says, "I feel like if I stretch a little farther here or hold this a little longer, something will open up or release more."

> Trust and listen to yourself.

How Do Muscles Get Strong

Muscles stay strong by using them. Muscles *get stronger* by using them more.

> For muscles to get stronger, we have to overload them. We have to put more demand on them than they are used to.

What this amounts to is that if you really want to strengthen a muscle . . . if you really, really want to get the most out of your time spent . . . then you have to work a muscle to at least about 80% of its maximum. In weight-lifting lingo, you have to fatigue the muscle.

Ugh—I hear a collective cry of anguish. That means that sorta painful, uncomfortable feeling we all (except for those weird few) hate. That means pushing ourselves. More cries of protest.

And then you leave the muscle alone and nature does the rest like putting a cake in the oven and leaving it there. It is during the "off" time that actual changes occur resulting in increased strength.

Unfortunately this need to fatigue muscles can be a problem when prescribing an exercise program. One size doesn't fit all when it comes to the amount of resistance required to build any individual's muscular strength.

Have you ever wondered why one exercise book says, "Do ten repetitions," and another one says, "Do this fifteen times." How do they decide on the right number? How do they know?

They don't know. They pick; they guess. This is where you come in. In the strengthening exercises, you need to do enough repetitions or hold the pose for enough time to make it hard for you, regardless of what number I pick. My number of repetitions or time may be above or below what you need. No need to kill yourself to start with but do make it a little hard and a little fatiguing because that's when the work gets done. If you're going to spend the time doing repetitions, do the extra ones or hold for a few seconds longer to get the fatigue feeling. That's when you build strength.

Building Strong Muscles In Two Ways

There are two ways muscles get stronger. Muscles increase in size, that is, the actual cross-sectional area of the muscle fibers increases (but don't worry, you won't bulk up doing any of the exercises in this book). The other way is muscles increase in functional efficiency—the coordination, number, and firing of the muscle units improves. Our bodies figure out how to use the muscle we have more effectively.

Or to put it in complex muscle kineseology jargon: "If frequent loads are administered to muscle tendon units in the moderate overload range, changes in external form and internal architecture occur in ways that allow them to better withstand the time-averaged increase in load." (Watkins, *Structure and Function of the Musculoskeletal System*, 1999)

How We Gain Flexibility

To build strength, we overload. To build flexibility, we overstretch.

Remember why we want flexibility. Tightness is what keeps us in our crooked positions. And we want our joints to reside somewhere in the middle of their ranges of motion, not maxed out to one side or the other.

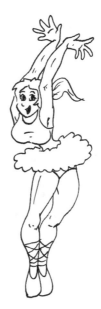

Our joints
need room
to move,
baby!

But there is a protective stretch-reflex mechanism in the body that tries to keep us from stretching. The body sees any stretching outside its normal range as a possible threat or danger and it clamps down by contracting the opposing muscle. It does this to prevent damage to vital joints. It's the body's way of saying, "Look, you haven't gone this far in a long time. I'm not sure whether you want to or if this is happening by accident. So I'm not going to let you do it because, until I hear otherwise, this seems like a mistake." The body is double-checking with us: "Do you really want to do this?"

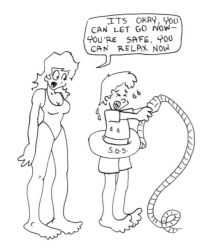

Stretching is the gradual process of convincing your muscles (physiologically) to release more. That's why gentle stretching, no bouncing, no sudden movements, works best.

Muscles consist of little muscle-unit segments called sarcomeres that are basically zippered together. If the sarcomeres are left in a shortened position (not stretched over long periods of time) they lose some of their unzipping ability. You can get it back but it takes time.

Flexibility is best achieved by stretching up to the level of discomfort, that is, close to the pain threshold. This is an art. And your flexibility can vary on any given day, with how warm you are, or with the time of day. How long should you hold or work a stretch? About thirty seconds is enough.

One of the keys to effective stretching is to control as many variables (other areas of the body) as possible, so that you get the stretch where you want it. That's why positioning is so crucial in the Posture Alignment exercises which follow.

And it's not just about stretching a muscle. We want to stretch our muscles in the correct directions that give us the space to allow our bodies to re-align themselves.

Muscle isn't the only thing that has to stretch and re-adapt, however. All our connective tissue—skin, fascia, tendons, ligaments— has to be slowly stretched and allowed to adapt too. All of this takes time.

> To build flexibility, we have to overstretch.

But enough talk, let's get on to the exercises . . .

CHAPTER 7

The Exercises

The beautiful motion is that which produces
the desired result with the least effort.

– Plato

Okay, here are the exercises—like recipes in a diet book. This is where we actually put what we've been talking about into practice.

First of all, don't be intimidated. There are lots of different menus and exercises. You won't be asked to do all of them; in fact, if you want you can start off doing only one or two exercises. All of the exercises help move you toward functional alignment. And remember—

> ## Anything you do will help.

In the first section of this chapter, the exercises are grouped into menus. First, there are several short menus that will introduce you to Posture Alignment. Next, there are remedial menus that address specific alterations in posture as diagnosed in Chapter 4. For variety two remedial menus, arbitrarily named #1 and #2, are given for each posture alteration category. You can do either one, both, or alternate between them.

For example, if your shoulders are rolled too far forward, you need to stretch open the front of your chest and shoulders, strengthen your back muscles, and realign your hips. There are two menus of exercises that address this problem. You can use both or either.

The sequence of the exercises in a given menu is important. Remember, we often have to first stretch open an area—gaining some space—before we can restore lost strength. Hence, you will get the most benefit by doing the exercises in the prescribed sequence.

After the remedial exercise menus, there are several overall alignment menus and some specialty menus.

The final two menus are easy. If you have trouble doing one of the regular menus or have significant health problems, you might want to skip to one of these. The first of the two easy menus can be done almost entirely while sitting in a chair. The second one can be done predominantly on the floor or while lying in bed.

Alongside each menu's name is given the number of exercises in the menu, the approximate time it takes to do the entire menu, and the page number where the menu begins.

On the menu pages themselves, a small picture of each exercise is given along with the exercise's name, and the page number where you can find a detailed description of that specific exercise. The number of repetitions to do, or the time to hold or stretch in the position is also listed.

For example, "20-40" means start by doing twenty repetitions and over time work your way up to forty. "15 seconds - 1 minute" means initially attempt to stretch or hold the position for fifteen seconds. Over time work your way up to doing it for a full minute.

The first few times you do a menu, you will need to refer back to the page on which each individual exercise is described to make sure you are doing them properly. Once you get the hang of it, you can just use the menu page.

List Of Posture Alignment Menus

An Introduction to Posture Alignment (3 exercises) 5 minutes - p. 111

If You Only Have Time For One (1 exercise) 1- 10 minutes - p. 111

Short Workout #1 (5 exercises) 16 minutes - p. 111
Short Workout #2 (5 exercises) 12 minutes -p. 112

Rounded Shoulders and Upper Back #1 (8 exercises) 20 minutes - p. 113
Rounded Shoulders and Upper Back #2 (11 exercises) 25 minutes - p. 114

Pelvis Tilted Forward #1 (11 exercises) 26 minutes - p. 115
Pelvis Tilted Forward #2 (13 exercises) 27 minutes - p. 116

Pelvis Tilted Backward #1 (12 exercises) 26 minutes - p. 117
Pelvis Tilted Backward #2 (15 exercises) 31 minutes - p. 118

Asymmetry of Shoulders and Hips—One Shoulder or Hip Higher or More Forward Than the Other #1 (13 exercises) 25 minutes - p. 119
Asymmetry of Shoulders and Hips—One Shoulder or Hip Higher or More Forward Than the Other #2 (12 exercises) 26 minutes - p. 120

Knee/Ankle/Foot #1 (15 exercises) 31 minutes - p. 121
Knee/Ankle/Foot #2 (15 exercises) 26 minutes - p. 122

Overall Alignment Workout #1 (16 exercises) 31 minutes - p. 123
Overall Alignment Workout #2 (22 exercises) 42 minutes - p. 124-125

Function Menu (exercises that strengthen muscles we use in day-to-day living) (5 exercises) 10 minutes - p. 126

Easy Menu #1 (can be done in a chair) (8 exercises) 18 minutes - p. 127
Easy Menu #2 (can be done on floor or modified for bed) (10 exercises) 18 minutes - p. 128

Choosing A Menu

Start off with the remedial menu appropriate for you. Or if you want a slower start, do one of the introductory or short menus for a few days to get a feel for the exercises and then progress to one of the remedial menus.

   Which remedial menu to use?

From your evaluation in Chapter 4, you might have one or two or more areas of your posture that need help. Some general guidelines are

• If you have asymmetry of shoulders and hips (one shoulder or hip higher or more forward than the other), use the "Asymmetry of Shoulders and Hips" menu first. Asymmetry takes precedence over any other postural problem. Until you correct or begin to correct this, it can be difficult to correct any other problem. Do either of the two "Asymmetry" menus until you have made significant progress in correcting this.

• The next priority is to correct your pelvis. If your hips are tilted forward or backward, address those areas first. If you have asymmetry of shoulders and hips, address them second. Try to be reasonably sure whether you have a level pelvis, a forward-tilted pelvis, or a backward-tilted pelvis since the exercises are somewhat different. You won't break anything or cause any harm by doing the wrong menu, but things simply won't correct as quickly. Do the pelvic menu appropriate for you until you begin to see and feel significant change.

• After several weeks you can begin to incorporate or alternate with the other menus, such as the Rolled Shoulders menu (rolled shoulders often go along with abnormal pelvic tilting).

• If you primarily have knee, ankle, or foot problems or rounded shoulders and otherwise are reasonably aligned, use the "Knee/Ankle/Foot" or "Rounded Shoulders" menus respectively.

• There is considerable overlap between the menus; they share many of the same exercises. If you have the time or have two or more problem areas, it is perfectly reasonable to intermesh two or more of the menus.

• These are guidelines: asymmetry first, pelvic tilting second followed by additional menus as needed. We are all different and correct at different rates. Hence, it is difficult to be much more specific than this. Part of the Posture Alignment process involves you, over time, becoming increasingly aware of your posture and for what needs to be corrected and how to do it. The menus and exercises are tools to do this.

How Often And For How Long To Do The Exercises

Every day would be ideal. Every other day is also good. Anything you do is going to help. Give the exercises as much time as you comfortably can without feeling too pressured. It is better to do less and keep doing it than to burn yourself out in a few days or even worse, make yourself feel guilty for not doing enough.

Maybe you can only do the exercises for five or ten minutes every other day. Pick one of the shorter menus and work on that. If you just try some of these exercises, you will feel the results. They will make you feel better and you will want to do them more.

The only caveat to all of this is that your progress may not be as quick if you don't do them frequently enough.

If you are reasonably faithful in doing the exercises, your body will begin to correct itself. You will feel your posture changing. You will feel more "lifted" and perhaps even get a little taller. Every few weeks take another look in the mirror and reevaluate. If you have corrected one area, then you can begin to correct another area.

If you are or become perfectly straight or close to it, you can use the "Overall Alignment" menus. It is okay for anyone to use them but, if your alignment is off, you'll be better off doing the remedial menus first.

Also, if any particular exercise is painful or you absolutely can't do it for any reason, look for one of the easier alternatives in the exercise portion of this chapter, or drop that exercise for now and try to come back to it at a later time.

Will These Exercises Correct All Of My Problems?

Maybe. It all depends. For some people who are reasonably active and only a little off in their alignment, results can be quick and dramatic. Others, who are very stiff, may not ever become completely straight. But these exercises, depending on the time you spend and the diligence you apply in doing them correctly, will move you strongly in the direction of postural alignment.

> Any movement toward postural alignment helps.

Also, a great variety of people will read a book; some may be very active to begin with, others may not have done anything in a long time. That's where you come in. You may have to adjust the number of repetitions and the time you hold some of the stretches to match your level of fitness or un-fitness to optimize their benefit for you.

Am I personally in perfect alignment? No—but I'm close. And there is a night-and-day difference between how I look, feel, and move now compared to the way I was before.

How Long Does It Take To Correct Things?

It depends on your alignment to begin with and how often you do the exercises. I'd be lying if I said it occurs overnight. It takes weeks, months, or even years. Remember though, just a little change may be enough to get rid of a nagging pain, or markedly improve your appearance or function.

You should feel a difference the *first time* you do one of the menus. They should bring your body back toward functional alignment. You should feel different and better. Then, usually within minutes, you will slowly revert back to your old posture. But with each time you do the exercises, you will stay aligned for a longer period of time.

Gains are also often made in starts and stops. Just because things don't immediately correct completely doesn't mean things aren't going on beneath the surface. You might go along for a while and not feel much and then suddenly you will see and feel a noticeable change in your alignment.

> The return to postural alignment always correlates with an increase in energy. You will feel you want to and are physically able to do more.

The Exercises

Following the menu section, exercises are grouped according to the muscles or area of the body they address. For example, all exercises that primarily strengthen the calf muscles are grouped together. This is where you will go to learn the individual exercises for your menu, and also where you can go to learn additional, complementary exercises.

If you know a significant part of your problem is lack of range of motion in your shoulders, you can find a whole series of exercises in this a la carte section that address this problem. The exercise section begins on page 129.

So many exercises shown in exercise books are boring or next to impossible to do correctly. I've only picked the exercises that I personally like and that are relatively easy to do with correct alignment. For each exercise group, there is usually a main exercise, that is, a middle-of-the-road exercise that most people should be able to do and is challenging enough to give results. This main exercise is also often the one used in the exercise menus.

If you are unable to do any specific exercise in a menu correctly for any reason, you can also flip back to this section and find an alternative exercise that is less demanding and addresses the same muscles. Ideally, after a period of time doing the milder exercise, you should be able to move back to the exercise listed in the menu.

Alternative exercises address the same muscle groups in slightly different ways. I would encourage you to try all of them at some point. They all complement each other. And sometimes, when one exercise isn't getting the job done, a slightly different version will produce results.

For most people, however, doing the exercises listed in the menus will be all you need to start.

I know you want to get started but there are several other key points about the exercises.

Read The Exercise Directions Carefully

You may look at some of the exercise pictures and say, "Oh, yeah, I can do that," and not bother reading the description carefully. Wait! There are often one or two key points that differ from how you may be used to doing a similar exercise. These differences are significant and are what makes Posture Alignment work.

You've come this far in changing your thinking on posture—so trust me a little farther and read the directions carefully so that you get maximum benefit.

Do The Exercises With Correct Alignment

Correct positioning of your body as stated in the instructions for the exercises is the key factor in making them do their job. This is what makes them different from normal exercises. You can't just haphazardly go through the motions and expect to get maximal results.

> If you aren't doing the exercises with correct alignment, you won't get maximum benefit.

I recognize initially that it may be hard to initially achieve perfect alignment. I mean that's why you're doing this program to begin with, right? But you have to make a continual effort to be conscious of your alignment. At first, perhaps your alignment may be just a rough approximation. Don't give up. Each time you do the exercises you will be able to align yourself more accurately.

Also while doing the exercises, particularly the gravity exercises (which I will tell you about in a moment), you may tend to fall out of correct alignment. Be vigilant. Remember how we talked about compensation? Your body will want to compensate. It will be up to its old tricks. It may not want to use that new muscle or stretch where it hasn't been stretching.

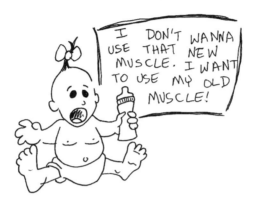

The fact that we fall out of alignment means things are working. It means we are giving a new stimulus and direction to our bodies. So if your body creeps out of correct alignment during an exercise then readjust. Part of the Posture Alignment process is to place ourselves in correct alignment as much as possible until a shift occurs and that becomes our new home.

The following key points on alignment apply to all the exercises unless stated otherwise:

• Feet should be hip-width apart.

• Feet should point straight ahead. Watch this one—they will want to turn in or out.

• Shoulders should be back. To remind yourself of correct shoulder positioning think of bringing your shoulders first up toward your ears, then back, and then relaxing them down. "Shoulders up, back, and then down."

• Hips should be evenly positioned. Particularly on exercises where you are lying on the floor or sitting, you should feel your weight evenly distributed on both hips or both sitting bones. Neither side should be cocked out to the side.

• Back should be in a neutral position—not overly arched or overly flat. As we've discussed, our backs aren't straight lines; they have natural curves to them. As much as possible we want to reinforce these natural curves.

• Do the exercises barefoot if possible. This helps strengthen and align the muscles in the feet and calves.

> One more time! If you aren't doing the
> exercises with correct alignment,
> you won't get the maximum benefit.

Here are several other suggestions.

• Use a small timer to time how long you are to hold each exercise. This is far easier and more effective than watching a clock or just guessing.

• If possible, do the exercises in front of a large wall mirror. This helps to assure correct positioning. We often think we are straight when we are not.

• Breathe! There is a tendency to want to hold your breath while stretching or exerting yourself. This deprives you of much-needed oxygen at exactly the time you need it most. So don't hold your breath, instead breath normally and deeply.

• After you've been doing the exercises for some time, go back and reread the instructions. You will pick up some fine points you may not have been able to fully understand until you did the exercises for a while.

• Do the exercises as prescribed, but if after doing them the allotted time you feel an area of tightness or feel you would benefit by altering your position slightly, go for it. Our bodies often tell us what we need to do.

Three Categories Of Exercises

The exercises generally fall into three categories: stretching, strengthening, and gravity or alignment exercises.

In **stretching exercises**, we are stretching tight muscles, tendons, and connective tissue, opening up space, and extending and maintaining our range of motion. One muscle can't get stronger until the opposing muscle lets go some. These exercises work on getting key areas to let go.

One key to effective stretching is to isolate the muscle you want to stretch. These exercises attempt to position your body so that you get the stretch where you are supposed to. But you need to follow the instructions carefully, and be vigilant about not bending your body in other areas to alleviate the stretch.

To maximize our time and effort in stretching, we need to stretch in a way that approaches our limits. Not until it hurts, but close—we need to feel a stretch. Er . . . that's why it's called stretching. Don't bounce. Hold and work the stretch for around thirty to sixty seconds.

Strengthening exercises work on strengthening weak muscle groups and bringing them into balance and alignment.

Remember, muscles get stronger by making them do more work than they are accustomed to. For a muscle to actually gain in strength, we have to push it to fatigue. *It has to be hard and hurt a little and be tiring.* Otherwise, we're just going through the motions. We will get some benefits but we certainly won't be maximizing the results we get.

This is where you may have to calibrate things more precisely for yourself. If and when one of the initial or primary exercises becomes too easy, that is, you have to do too many reps to feel anything, you may need to move on to a more demanding alternative in the exercise section. That way you don't have to do a million repetitions to get fatigued.

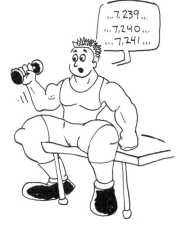

Also, on some of the exercises, you could use ankle or wrist weights or light dumbbells to make it harder and so that you don't need to do so many repetitions. But don't sacrifice alignment and correct form to try and progress too quickly.

Gravity (or alignment) exercises are the ones you may be the least familiar with. In these exercises we allow gravity and the weight of our own bodies to restore correct alignment. These are more passive exercises where we basically put ourselves into correct alignment, or as close to it as possible, and let our muscles slowly adjust to accommodate that position.

> The gravity exercises are the ones that do
> the real work of Posture Alignment.
> But they take time to do their job.

You may look at the gravity exercises and say, "Jeez, I can do that," or think they are for older, more disabled individuals than yourself. Don't be deceived, particularly you macho guys (or gals). This isn't about proving yourself or competing or anything like that; it is about getting back into functional alignment so that we can compete and prove ourselves (if that's your thing) at even higher levels.

An example of a gravity exercise is lying on our back with both your legs up on a block or chair (Astronaut - page 142). The longer you stay in this position, the more your lower back and hips settle into the ground and reposition themselves.

As stated before, if we try to forcibly correct our posture, it doesn't work. Our bodies immediately compensate or our stretch reflexes kick in to prevent us. So we have to kind of sneak up on it, like gently leading a horse to water and all that. The gravity exercises do this.

When doing the gravity exercises, at first, and for varying lengths of time, our muscles can hold out against correct alignment. Eventually, usually over several minutes, they start to let go and release. You will feel tiny micro-movements in your hips and shoulders and back. This is the Posture Alignment method working. Also, often after the first few minutes as our bodies begin to readjust, our alignment tends to alter. We may find our feet rolling outward or feel a tendency to lean to one side or the other. Be ready for this and readjust.

The more time you can spend in any of the gravity exercise positions while staying vigilant with your alignment, the faster the results.

> Give the gravity exercises time to do their work.

The gravity exercises also provide you with a perfect time to ask yourself some questions.

> Why doesn't the weight feel equal on both of my sitting bones?
> Why does one foot want to flare out while the other
> one remains straight ahead?
> Why does it feel tight on one side of my back and not the other?

And you and I will come up with all sorts of explanations in our heads—old injuries, family history, our bodies are unique, etc,—but 99.9% of the time the real reasons are weakness of certain muscles, tightness of others, and overall imbalance.

One final thing: gravity exercises can generally be done for as long as you like. Many of them can be done while watching TV or reading a book. Time spent in any of gravity exercises is like money in the bank.

What If The Exercises Don't Seem To Be Working?

Give them time. We are all a little different.

First, remember the initial signs of your posture changing can be subtle: a slight transfer in weight, less tension in one area, using a muscle you don't usually use, a different feeling when walking down stairs. Any of these things and countless more are signs of changes occurring in your alignment.

If you don't feel you are getting results, check the following things:

• Make sure you are consciously doing the exercises with correct alignment. Focus on what you are doing. Don't just schlump your way through them.

• On the strengthening exercises, make sure you are doing enough repetitions or holding the poses long enough with correct alignment to fatigue yourself. This is what builds strength where you need it.

• On the stretching exercises, make sure you are stretching at or close to your limits. Again, don't just go through the motions.

• Give the gravity exercises time to work. Don't cheat yourself out of their benefits.

• Sometimes you may not be doing the exercises often enough to overcome what is going on during the rest of your day. Consider doing them more often.

• If you still don't feel much change, consider re-evaluating what you read and saw in Chapter 4.

One More Time

> Anything you do will help.

Don't beat yourself up on how much or how little you decide to do. This is no competition. It's not an all-or-nothing proposition. Anything you do can only help. But do something.

How To Bend Forward Without Hurting Yourself

What often hurts or injures us when we bend forward is excessive rounding of our lower backs, along with not having enough core strength to support ourselves. This puts undo strain on our lower backs.

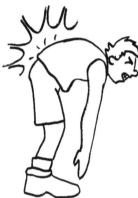

   Sure, you can bend your knees and squat anytime you bend, but let's learn to bend forward without excessively rounding our lower backs.

   Look at the Cats and Dogs exercise (page 167). Get down on the floor and practice the dog portion where you increase the arch in your back and lift your rear end slightly.

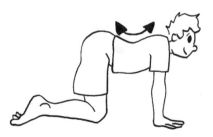

   This is the movement you want to create with your pelvis when you bend forward. You want to keep your low back flat or a slight arch with you bend forward.

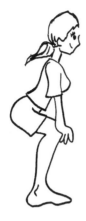

Stand up straight. While keeping your abdominal muscles in, re-create the dog arch in your back and bend forward slightly, placing your hands on your knees. Don't go any farther for now. Go up and down a few times maintaining the arch in your back.

Now you're ready to go a little deeper. Stand a few feet from a table, go into your dog arch, and then bend forward placing your hands on the table. Come back up.

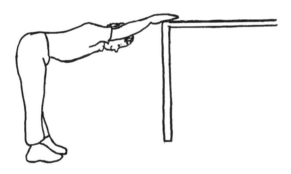

See how easy that is. It is now only a matter of increasing your abdominal strength (the Abdominal exercises on page 129 will help) and flexibility to go farther. The basic alignment principle remains the same however for all yoga-type forward bends, whether standing up or sitting on the floor.

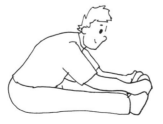

The Exercise Menus

An Introduction to Posture Alignment   Total Time: 5 minutes

1. Table Stretch
1 minute
Page 140
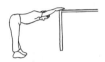

3. Stair Drop
2 minutes
Page 148

2. Floor Sit
2 minutes
Page 141
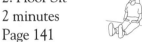

If You Only Have Time For One. Try one of these.

Table Stretch
1 minute
Page 140
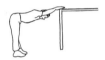

Stair Drop
2 minutes
Page 148

Groin Stretch
5 minutes each side
Page 155

Short Workout #1   Total Time: 16 minutes

1. Cats and Dogs
10 cycles
Page 167

4. Stair Drop
2 - 3 minutes
Page 148

2. Floor Twist
1 minute each side
Page 182

5. Groin Stretch
5 minutes each side
Page 155

3. Face the Wall
1- 3 minutes
Page 143
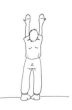

Short Workout #2   Total Time: 12 minutes

1. Arm Circles
30 circles each direction
Page 172

4. Face Plant
2-5 minutes
Page 143

2. Astronaut
5 minutes
Page 142

5. Wall Bench
15 seconds - 2 minutes
Page 164

3. Chair Twist
1 minute each side
Page 183

Rounded Shoulders and Upper Back #1   Total Time: 20 minutes

What's going on
- Tightness of muscles in front of chest and shoulders
- Relative weakness of muscles in back of shoulders and in upper back
- Pelvis not aligned

What we need to do
- Stretch out front of chest and shoulders
- Strengthen muscles in upper back and between shoulder blades
- Reintroduce full range of motion to shoulders
- Align pelvis

MENUS

1. Arm Circles
30 circles each direction
Page 172

5. Stair Drop
(or Slant Board)
2-3 minutes (5-10 minutes)
Page 148 (Page 149)

2. Table Stretch
1 minute
Page 140

6. Imaginary Chair
15 - 60 seconds X 2
Page 163

3. Shoulder Squeezes
and Overheads on Floor
20 reps
Page 178

7. Floor Sit
2 minutes
Page 141

4. Face the Wall
1- 3 minutes
Page 143

8. Groin Stretch
5 minutes each side
Page 155

Rounded Shoulders and Upper Back #2   Total Time: 25 minutes

1. Arm Circles
30 circles each direction
Page 172

2. Elbow Curls
20 curls
Page 173

3. Backstroke
5 each arm forward
then backward
Page 175

4. Overhead Extension
30 seconds - 1 minute
Page 140

5. Standing Shoulder
Squeezes
20 squeezes
Page 176

6. Face Plant
2-5 minutes
Page 143

7. Angel Arms
10 cycles
Page 174

8. Stair Drop
(or Slant Board)
2-3 minutes
(5-10 minutes)
Page 148 (Page 149)

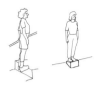

9. Shoulder Squeezes
and Overheads in Astronaut
10 of each
Page 178

10. Sitting and Standing
Work up to 20 times
Page 162

11. Groin Stretch
5 minutes each side
Page 155

Pelvis Tilted Forward #1   Total Time: 26 minutes

What's going on
- Muscles in front of groins too tight
- Tight quads and hamstrings
- Tight low back muscles
- Weak abdominal muscles

What we need to do
- Stretch out muscles in front of hips
- Stretch quads, hamstrings, and low back muscles
- Strengthen abdominal muscles
- Restore range of motion back to pelvis

1. Astronaut
5 minutes
Page 142

7. Abdominal Crunches
at Wall
20-50
Page 129

2. Cats and Dogs
10 cycles
Page 167

8. Foot Clock and Points
10-30 each direction each
foot; 10-20 points
Page 139

3. Child's Pose
30 seconds - 1 minute
Page 133

9. Toe Raises (3 part)
10-20 each position
Page 137

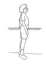

4. Hamstring Stretch
at Corner
30 seconds each side
Page 151

10. Wall Bench
15 seconds - 2 minutes
Page 164

5. Japanese Sitting Pose
30 seconds - 1 minute
Page 171

11. Groin Stretch
5 minutes each side
Page 155

6. Leg to Chest
30 seconds each side
Page 156

Pelvis Tilted Forward #2   Total Time: 27 minutes

1. Cats and Dogs
10 cycles
Page 167

2. Downward Dog
30 seconds
Page 132

3. Hamstring Stretch
with Strap
15 seconds each position
each leg
Page 150

4. Leg to Chest
30 seconds each side
Page 156

5. Standing Bent-Knee
Chair Twist
1 minute each side
Page 184

6. Abdominal Crunches
at Wall
20-50
Page 129

7. Hip Stretch at Wall
30 seconds each side
Page 153

8. Japanese Sitting Pose
30 seconds - 1 minute
Page 171

9. Child's Pose
30 seconds - 1 minute
Page 133

10. Toe Raises (3 part)
10-20 each position
Page 137

11. Stair Drop
(or Slant Board)
2-3 minutes
(5-10 minutes)
Page 148 (Page 149)

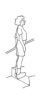

12. Imaginary Chair
15 - 60 seconds X 2
Page 163

13. Groin Stretch
5 minutes each side
Page 155

Pelvis Tilted Backward #1   Total Time: 26 minutes

What's going on
- Muscles which flex our thighs are weak
- Other muscles surrounding pelvis including glutes often weak
- Hamstrings can be tight
- Low back muscles may be weak

What we need to do
- Stretch hamstrings
- Strengthen muscles in front of thighs and surrounding pelvis
- Restore range of motion back to pelvis

1. Arm Circles
30 circles each direction
Page 172

2. Table Stretch
1 minute
Page 140

3. Cats and Dogs
10 cycles
Page 167

4. Hamstring Stretch
with Strap
15 seconds each
position each leg
Page 150

5. Leg Lifts
20-40 each side
Page 163

6. Foot Clock and Points
10-30 each direction each
foot;10-20 points
Page 139

7. Bridge Lift
5-20 lifts
Page 144

8. Face the Wall
1- 3 minutes
Page 143

9. Pillow Squeezes
on Chair
20-40 squeezes
Page 160

10. Sitting and
Standing
10 - 20 times
Page 162

Look Ma, no hands!

11. Floor Sit
2 minutes
Page 141

12. Groin Stretch
5 minutes each side
Page 155

Pelvis Tilted Backward #2   Total Time: 31 minutes

1. Arm Circles
30 circles each direction
Page 172

2. Elbow Curls
20 curls
Page 173

3. Cats and Dogs
10 cycles
Page 167

4. Face Plant
2-5 minutes
Page 143

5. Pushups
10-20
Page 177

6. Airplane
15-30 seconds X 2
Page 177

7. Locust Leg Lifts
15 seconds each
side X 2
Page 145

8. Hamstring Stretch
at Wall
30 seconds
Page 151

9. Pillow Squeezes on Chair
20-40 squeezes
Page 160

10. Toe Raises (3 part)
10-20 each position
Page 137

11. Sitting and Standing
10 - 20 times
Page 162

12. Standing Side
Leg Lifts
10-20 each side
Page 166

13. Stair Drop
(or Slant Board)
2-3 minutes
(5-10 minutes)
Page 148 (Page 149)

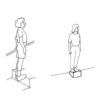

14. Wall Bench
15 seconds - 2 minutes
Page 164

15. Groin Stretch
5 minutes each side
Page 155

Asymmetry of Shoulders and Hips—One Shoulder or Hip Higher or More Forward Than the Other #1   Total Time: 25 minutes

What's going on
- Imbalance of muscle strength and flexibility in our shoulders, backs, and pelvis
- Muscles on one side of the chest and upper back are tight while those on other side are relatively weak and stretched
- Muscles on one side of the pelvis, hips, and flanks are tight while those on the other side are relatively weak and stretched

What we need to do
- Stretch muscles surrounding shoulders, back, and pelvis
- Align and symmetrically strengthen the same areas

MENUS

1. Cats and Dogs
10 cycles
Page 167

2. Table Stretch
1 minute
Page 140

3. Hamstring Stretch at Corner
30 seconds each side
Page 151

4. Floor Twist
1 minute each side
Page 182

5. Crocodile Twist
30 seconds each side
Page 183

6. Triangle at the Wall
15 - 30 seconds each side
Page 180

7. Face the Wall
1- 3 minutes
Page 143

8. Crossover Leg Stretch
30 seconds each side
Page 154

9. Hip Stretch at Wall
30 seconds each side
Page 153

10. Stair Drop
2-3 minutes
Page 148

11. Imaginary Chair
15 - 60 seconds X 2
Page 163

12. Floor Sit
2 minutes
Page 141

13. Groin Stretch
5 minutes each side
Page 155

Asymmetry of Shoulders and Hips—One Shoulder or Hip Higher or More Forward Than the Other #2   Total Time: 26 minutes

1. Arm circles
30 circles each direction
Page 172

2. Cats and Dogs
10 cycles
Page 167

3. Table Stretch
1 minute
Page 140

4. Hamstring Stretch
with Strap
15 seconds each
position each leg
Page 150

5. Floor Twist
1 minute each side
Page 182

6. Standing Quad Stretch
30 seconds each side
Page 170

7. Child's Pose
30 seconds - 1 minute
Page 133

8. Chair Twist
1 minute each side
Page 183

9. Standing Bent-Knee
Chair Twist
1 minute each side
Page 184

10. Floor Sit
2 minutes
Page 141

11. Wall Bench
15 seconds - 2 minutes
Page 164

12. Groin Stretch
5 minutes each side
Page 155

Knee/Ankle/Foot #1   Total Time: 31 minutes

What's going on
- Imbalance of muscle flexibility, strength, and alignment in pelvis, thigh, or calf muscles or some combination of them

What we need to do
- Stretch all major muscle groups surrounding pelvis and lower extremities
- Symmetrically strengthen individual muscle groups

MENUS

1. Cats and Dogs
10 cycles
Page 167

2. Face the Wall
1- 3 minutes
Page 143

3. Standing Shoulder Squeezes
20 squeezes
Page 176

4. Floor Twist
1 minute each side
Page 182

5. Crossover Leg Stretch
30 seconds each side
Page 154

6. Frog
1 minute
Page 158

7. Hip Stretch at Wall
30 seconds each side
Page 153

8. Foot Clock and Points
10-30 each direction each foot;10-20 points
Page 139

9. Pillow Squeezes on Chair
20-40 squeezes
Page 160

10. Hamstring Stretch at Corner
30 seconds each side
Page 151
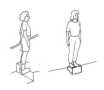

11. Stair Drop
(or Slant Board)
2-3 minutes
(5-10 minutes)
Page 148 (Page 149)

12. Toe raises (3 part)
10-20 each position
Page 137

13. Standing Side Leg Lifts
10-20 each side
Page 166

14. Wall Bench
15 seconds - 2 minutes
Page 164

15. Groin Stretch
5 minutes each side
Page 155

Knee/Ankle/Foot #2   Total Time: 26 minutes

1. Arm Circles
30 circles each direction
Page 172

9. Standing Quad Stretch
30 seconds each side
Page 170

2. Cats and Dogs
10 cycles
Page 167

10. Standing Bent-Knee
Chair Twist
1 minute each side
Page 184

3. Hamstring Stretch
with Strap
15 seconds each
position each leg
Page 150

11. Stair Drop
(or Slant Board)
2-3 minutes
(5-10 minutes)
Page 148 (Page 149)
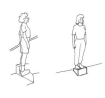

4. Leg to Chest
30 seconds each side
Page 156

12. Standing Toe Raises
10 times
Page 138

5. Face Plant
2-5 minutes
Page 143

13. Imaginary Chair
15 - 60 seconds X 2
Page 163

6. Pillow Squeezes
on Floor
20 -40 squeezes
Page 160

14. Floor Sit
2 minutes
Page 141

7. Side-Lying Leg Lifts
10-20 each side
Page 166
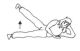

15. Tree Pose
1 minute each side
Page 134

8. Reverse Frog at Wall
1-3 minutes
Page 159

Overall Alignment Workout #1   Total Time: 31 minutes

1. Arm circles
30 circles each direction
Page 172

2. Elbow Curls
20 curls
Page 173

3. Overhead Extension
30 seconds - 1 minute
Page 140

4. Table Stretch
1 minute
Page 140

5. Cats and Dogs
10 cycles
Page 167

6. Downward Dog
30 seconds
Page 132

7. Hamstring Stretch
with Strap
15 seconds each
position each leg
Page 150

8. Bridge Lift
5-20 lifts
Page 144

9. Floor Twist
1 minute each side
Page 182

10. Imaginary Chair
15 - 60 seconds X 2
Page 163

11. Toe Raises (3 part)
10-20 each position
Page 137
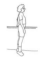

12. Stair Drop
(or Slant Board)
2-3 minutes
(5-10 minutes)
Page 148 (Page 149)

13. Triangle
30 seconds each side
Page 180

14. Wide-Leg Forward Bend
30 seconds
Page 152

15. Standing Bent-Knee
Chair Twist
1 minute each side
Page 184

16. Groin Stretch
5 minutes each side
Page 155
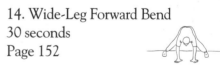

MENUS

Overall Alignment Workout #2   Total Time: 42 minutes

1. Arm Circles
30 circles each
direction
Page 172

2. Backstroke
5 each arm forward
then backward
Page 175

3. Overhead Extension
30 seconds - 1 minute
Page 140

4. Cats and Dogs
10 cycles
Page 167

5. Downward Dog
30 seconds
Page 132

6. Floor Twist
1 minute each side
Page 182

7. Crocodile Twist
30 seconds each side
Page 183

8. Frog
1 minute
Page 158

9. Crossover Leg Stretch
30 seconds each side
Page 154

10. Stair Drop
(or Slant Board)
2-3 minutes
(5-10 minutes)
Page 148 (Page 149)

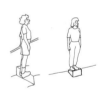

11. Hamstring Stretch
at Wall
30 seconds
Page 151

12. Single-Legged
Table Stretch
1 minute each side
Page 157

MENUS

13. Standing Toe Raises
10 times
Page 138

14. Standing Side
Leg Lifts
10-20 each side
Page 166

15. Wall Bench
15 seconds - 2 minutes
Page 164

16. Triangle
30 seconds each side
Page 180

17. Face Plant
2-5 minutes
Page 143

18. Airplane
15-30 seconds X 2
Page 177

19. Locust Leg Lifts
15 seconds each side X2
Page 145

20. Four-Part Abdominals
30 seconds each position
Page 130

21. Tree Pose
1 minute each side
Page 134

22. Groin Stretch
5 minutes each side
Page 155

Function Menu Total Time: 10 minutes
Five exercises that strengthen muscles we use in day-to-day living

1. Sitting and Standing
10 - 20 times
Page 162

2. Reaching Down Under
10 - 20 each side
Page 164

3. Getting Down
and Getting Up
10 each side
Page 165

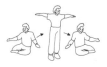

4. Standing Bent-Knee
Chair Twist
1 minute each side
Page 184

5. Pick-Ups
20 times
Page 165

Easy Menu #1   Total Time: 18 minutes
Can be done in a chair

1. Sitting Arm Circles
10-30 each direction
Page 173

2. Child's Pose on Chair
15 seconds -1 minute
Page 133

3. Chair Twist
30 seconds - 1 minute
each side
Page 183

4. Angel Arms on Chair
10 times
Page 174

5. Pillow Squeezes
on Chair
10-20 squeezes
Page 160

6. Seated Toe Raises
10-20 times
Page 137

7. Sitting and Standing
5 - 20 times
Page 162

Look Ma,
no hands!

8. Chair-Assisted
Balance
1 minute each side
Page 135

9. Astronaut
5 - 10 minutes
Page 142

Easy Menu #2   Total Time: 18 minutes
Can be done on floor or modified for bed

1. Pelvic Tilts
10 - 20 tilts
Page 167

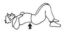

2. Angel Arms
10 times
Page 174

3. Shoulder Squeezes and
Overheads on Floor
10 of each
Page 178

4. Frog
30 seconds - 1 minute
Page 158

5. Glute Contractions
20 times
Page 154

6. Pillow Squeezes
on Floor
20 times
Page 160

7. Leg Lifts
10-30 each side
page 163

8. Floor Twist
1 minute each side
Page 182

9. Abdominal Crunches
(or Contractions)
10-20
Page 129 (Page 130)

10. Legs Up Wall
1- 5 minutes
Page 148

Groups of Exercises

ABDOMINAL EXERCISES

These exercises strengthen the abdominal muscles.

ABDOMINAL CRUNCHES AT WALL

Lie on your back with your feet against a wall with your knees and legs forming a

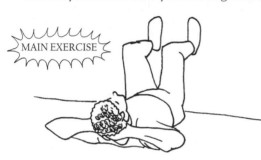

MAIN EXERCISE

ninety-degree angle with the rest of your body. Place your hands behind your head, gently clenching your fingers. Let your elbows relax down toward the floor. Now lift your head, neck, and shoulders *upward* toward the ceiling. Your head and neck only need to come off the floor about six inches. You want to lift upward, not forward toward your toes. Hold for a second and relax completely back down.

Do twenty, gradually working your way up to fifty over time.

Once you get the hang of this, you may also try to do some of your reps lifting slightly to the sides, that is, to the right and left working the side abdominals.

ABDOMINAL CRUNCHES

Lie on your back with your knees bent and your feet flat on the floor. Place your hands behind your head, gently clenching your fingers. Let your elbows relax down toward the floor. Now lift your head, neck, and shoulders *upward* toward the ceiling. Your head and neck only need to come off the floor about six inches. Hold for a second and then relax completely back down. You should feel this in your abdomen. The key is to not bend forward toward your toes as in a traditional sit-up but instead to lift upward. Keeping your gaze on the ceiling while doing this exercise may help remind you of this.

Do twenty gradually working your way up to fifty over time.

Once you get the hang of this, you may also try to do some of your reps lifting slightly to the sides, that is, to the right and left working the side abdominals.

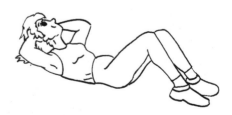

SIMPLE ABDOMINAL CONTRACTIONS

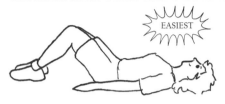

This is a milder abdominal workout. Sometimes it is difficult at first to isolate a muscle and then make the connection in your mind on how to get it to contract. This exercise helps. Lie on your back with your knees bent. Place your hands on your abdomen on either side of your navel. Now gently contract your abdominal muscles for a second. You should feet them tighten beneath your hands. Work on getting only your abdominal muscles to contract without your hip or back muscles doing any work.

Do ten, working when your way up to twenty, and eventually progress to the Abdominal Crunches exercises.

FOUR-PART ABDOMINALS

This is a four-part exercise. These can be challenging, which means *hard*, so make sure you listen to your own body and capability.

1. Plank Pose

Lie on the floor on your stomach. Gently clench your hands together on the floor beneath your head. Now lift your body up, supporting your weight on your elbows and toes. Your legs are straight. You want your body to be in a straight line (like a plank) neither sagging toward the floor nor with your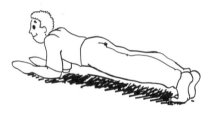
bottom or back lifting too high in the air. Focus on using your abdominal muscles to hold you in this position rather than your arms or shoulders.

At first you may only be able to hold for a few seconds. Work your way up to holding for thirty seconds, making sure that you don't sacrifice correct form.

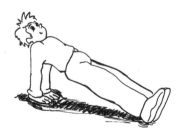

2. Reverse Plank

Sit on the floor with your legs extended and your feet together. Place your hands behind you near your waist with your fingers pointing toward your toes. Now lift up, supporting your weight on your hands and your heels. Once again, you want your body to be as straight as possible and not sagging toward the floor. Your head and neck are relaxed.

Work your way up to holding for thirty seconds.

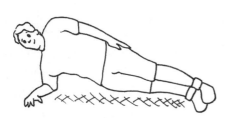

3 and 4. Side Abdominals

Lie on your right side. Your right elbow is on the floor beneath your head with your forearm and hand at a ninety-degree angle to your body and extending away from you with your palm down. Place your left foot on top of your right foot. If having one foot on top of the other is terribly uncomfortable, you can place your left foot on the floor just over the instep of your right foot.

Now lift up, supporting your weight on the side of your right foot and your right elbow and forearm. Again, you want to work on forming a nice straight line with the side of your body and not sag toward the floor. Concentrate on lifting with your right abdominal muscles.

Hold for a few seconds, working your way up to holding for thirty seconds. Repeat the exercise lying on your left side.

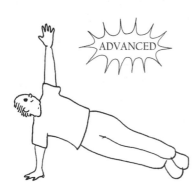

Variation: Lift up supporting your weight on your hand instead of your elbow and forearm. Balance becomes slightly more of a problem. Again, make sure you concentrate on forming a nice straight line with your entire body and lifting with your side abdominal muscles.

BACK STRETCHES

These exercises stretch and elongate the muscles in the back and along our spine.

DOWNWARD DOG

This is a classic yoga pose. Some yoga teachers say that if you do only one yoga exercise, this is the one to do. It stretches out the entire back of the body including the lower back and hamstrings. Get on the floor on your hands and knees. Your hands are directly under your shoulders, your knees are hip-width apart. Now, while leaving your hands and feet where they are, slowly push yourself up, lifting your bottom high in the air so that your body forms a triangle. Your hands are evenly spaced with your fingers pointing forward; your feet are hip-width apart with your toes pointing forward. Your back should be straight, that is, not sagging toward the floor nor overly lifting or arching upward. This can be difficult if you aren't used to it. Ideally, you want your weight evenly balanced between your hands and feet. If you can get your heels to the ground, that's great; if not, don't worry about it but keep your feet pointing straight ahead. Focus on lifting your rear end *up* and *back*.

Hold for fifteen to thirty seconds.

Alternative: If you can't do the whole pose, that's okay. Instead, just get down on your hands and knees (with feet and hands pointing straight ahead) and push up in any manner so that your weight is on your hands and feet. Don't worry initially about how straight things your back is. Just get the feel of supporting yourself on your hands and feet. Doing this even for a few seconds begins to strengthen muscles and provides a needed stretch to the back of your body.

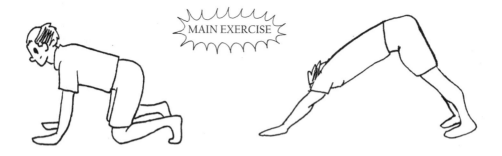

MAIN EXERCISE

CHILD'S POSE

This is a classic yoga relaxation pose, but initially it might not feel so relaxing if your lower back and hamstrings are tight. Sit on the floor Japanese style with your knees bent and your legs underneath you so that you are sitting on your heels. Try to keep both thighs pointing straight ahead. If this is terribly uncomfortable, you can modify the position by putting a small pillow under your bottom. If it is painful for your feet, put a small towel under your feet. Often we are tight in these areas, and it takes time for them to stretch out. Now, roll your body forward so that your chest is on or close to your thighs. Allow your hands to relax down at your sides. Your forehead rests gently on the floor. If your forehead can't touch the floor, you

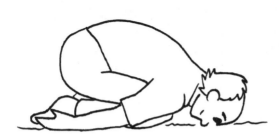

can use another small pillow to support it. You don't want it dangling in the air and causing more tension in your neck and back.

Stay in this position for thirty seconds to one minute or longer allowing your entire back to stretch and relax.

CHILD'S POSE ON CHAIR

Sit upright on a hard-bottomed chair. Your feet should be shoulder-width apart and pointing straight ahead. Place a pillow or cushion on your lap. Now, allow your upper body to fold and relax forward so that your chest lies on the pillow close to your thighs. You want to relax and let go in this pose, so make sure you have the right sized pillow. No tension; no holding on. Let your head, shoulders, and arms droop forward.

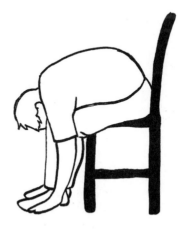

Relax in this pose for thirty seconds to one minute.

BALANCING ACTS

These exercises develop strength and coordination throughout the entire body particularly strengthening the muscles around the ankles, knees, and hips.

• It's the wobbling back and forth, the quivering legs, and the losing your balance that makes you stronger. The fact that you can't balance is not the point; the point is to try to balance.

> Anytime you are trying to balance you are
> gaining the strength and coordination
> to get better at balancing.

• Practice balancing on both sides. Invariably most people are better at balancing on one side than the other. Both sides have to be reminded to carry their full share of the load.

• One of the keys to balancing is to lock your supporting leg. Keep the supporting leg straight by activating the muscles in your quadriceps on that side.

• As a teacher once told me, all the variations of balancing on one leg (the various arm and leg movements) are just so much foo-foo. They are all just tricks and distractions to get you to balance, which is how the real strength develops.

TREE POSE

This is a classic yoga posture. Stand in the middle of the room. Lock your left leg so that your knee is straight. Bend your right leg and place your right foot on the inside of your left thigh. You may only be able to get it up to your knee or perhaps to your calf at first. This is fine. Place your hands in the center of your chest in "prayer" position. Let your shoulders relax down. Try to work on rotating your right knee outward, that is, away from the center of your body.

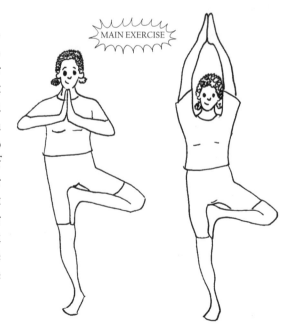

MAIN EXERCISE

EXERCISES

Practice this pose for one minute. If you lose your balance, try again until the whole minute is up. Repeat on the other side.

Once you are able to stand for a full minute without falling, practice raising your hands together above your head with your index fingers together and the rest of your fingers crossed. Progress until you are able to do this for one minute.

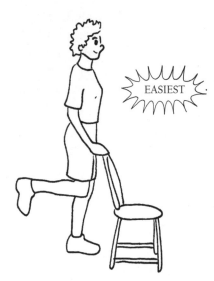

EASIEST

CHAIR-ASSISTED BALANCE

Stand next to a chair holding onto the back of the chair with one hand. Lift your right foot off the ground bending your knee backward. Lock the supporting leg. Your standing foot points straight ahead.

Stand for fifteen seconds working up to one minute. Repeat on the other side.

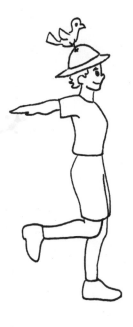

CHAIR-FREE BALANCE

When you are able to stand on one leg using a chair for support for a full minute, practice releasing your hand from the chair eventually moving the chair out of the way.

Practice for one minute on each side, If you lose your balance, try again until the minute is up. Work your way up so you are able to balance on one foot for one minute on each side.

WARRIOR THREE POSE

This is another, more advanced yoga balance pose. Stand with your feet together. Clasp your hands above your head with your index fingers straight and the rest of your fingers clenched together. Your arms should be straight with your biceps close to your ears. Step your right foot out in front of you, moving your weight onto your right foot and pointing your left foot behind you. Your right foot points straight ahead. Now, lean forward with your entire body, simultaneously bending forward with your arms and trunk while lifting your left hip and leg until your entire body is parallel to the ground. Reach toward the front wall with your hands, point your toes, and reach toward the back wall with your lifted foot. The key to the pose is to work on keeping your body straight by simply bending forward in one piece instead of jackknifing at your waist. Your arms remain alongside your ears and your face looks toward the ground.

Hold for ten seconds, then repeat on the other side. Work your way up to holding for thirty seconds.

This is a demanding pose. Make sure your supporting leg remains locked and the supporting foot remains pointing straight ahead. Level your hips so that a tray placed on your backside would not slide off to either side.

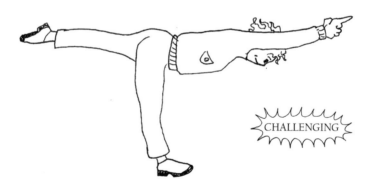

CHALLENGING

CALF EXERCISES

EXERCISES

These exercises predominately work on stretching, strengthening, and aligning the muscles in the calves.

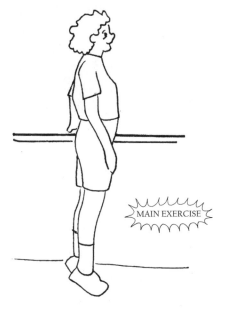

MAIN EXERCISE

TOE RAISES (3 part)

1. Stand up straight alongside something you can hold on to like a counter. Your feet are together and point straight ahead; try to keep your feet, ankles, knees, and thighs touching or close to it. Lift straight up onto your toes as high as you can, then slowly lower back down. Avoid leaning to one side or the other. Work up to twenty repetitions.

2. Turn your toes inward (pigeon-toed) so that your toes are touching and your heels are about six inches apart. Lift and lower, working up to twenty repetitions.

3. Turn your toes about six inches apart and place your heels together like a ballerina. Lift up on your toes and then lower. Work up to doing twenty of these.

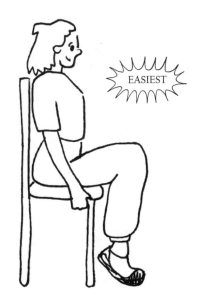

EASIEST

SEATED TOE RAISES

Sit on a hard-bottomed chair with your feet hip-width apart and pointing straight ahead. Your back is straight and your shoulders are back. While remaining seated, lift your heels off the floor so that you are up on your toes. Lift and stretch as high as you can while maintaining good alignment.

Do twenty of these.

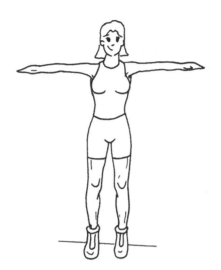

STANDING TOE RAISES

Stand in the center of the room with your feet straight ahead and hip-width apart. Raise your arms out to the side at shoulder level. Now, lift up on your toes. You're a bird. Hold for a few seconds and then gently lower your heels back down to the floor.

Repeat ten times.

IMAGINARY CHAIR ON TOES

Stand with your feet six inches apart and your toes pointing straight ahead. Extend your arms out in front of you at shoulder level with your palms down. Lift up onto your toes so that your weight is on your toes and the balls of your feet. *While remaining on your toes* and keeping your back straight and upright, lower yourself down as if you were sitting in an imaginary chair. At first you may only be able to go part way down.

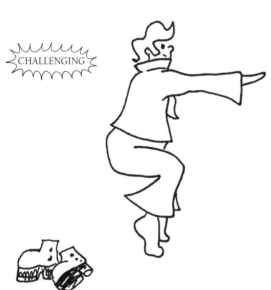

CHALLENGING

Hold for fifteen seconds. Then, while still staying up on your toes, first push yourself up and then release your heels down. Over time work on getting down far enough so that your thighs are parallel with the ground. Concentrate on lifting higher and higher up on your toes while keeping your back straight. Work up to holding for one minute.

FOOT CLOCK AND POINTS

Lie on your back. Bend your right leg, grasping hold of it with both hands behind the knee. Your left leg remains flat on the floor. Concentrate on keeping your right knee firmly fixed in your hands; you want the movement to come from your foot and ankle. Now circle your foot ten times to the right. Pretend your toes are the hands of a clock; make sure they stretch and reach every number on the clock. Then circle your foot ten times in the other direction. Next, point and flex your foot ten times. In this exercise, concentrate on stretching your foot and ankles as far as you can in all directions so that you begin to regain lost range-of-motion territory. Repeat on the other side.

Work up to doing thirty circles in each direction on both sides and twenty foot points.

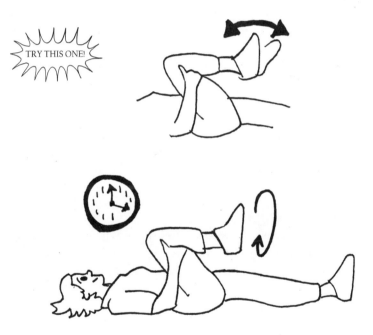

TRY THIS ONE!

CHEST AND SHOULDER OPENERS

These exercises open up, stretch, and align the muscles in the chest and shoulders.

TABLE STRETCH
This exercise counteracts the tendency to hunch and roll our shoulders forward. Find a table, desk, counter, or railing; something waist height works best. Your feet are hip-width apart and pointing straight ahead. Lean forward and rest your hands palms down on the table. You want your legs and your torso to form a ninety-degree angle. You may have to adjust your position to get it just right. Relax. Let your head fall forward between your shoulders and let your shoulders relax. Let gravity do the work. You should feel this exercise in your shoulders, upper back, and also possibly

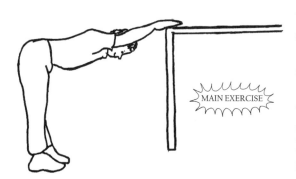

MAIN EXERCISE

in the hamstring area. Adjust your position so that you feel an appropriate stretch for you.

Hold for one minute and eventually two minutes.

As a variation, you can try turning your hands palms upward or as close as possible. Everything else remains the same. Relax and let go.

OVERHEAD EXTENSION
Stand with your feet pointing forward and hip-width apart. Clasp your fingers together and raise them over your head so that your palms point upward. Look upward toward the backs of your hands. Concentrate on trying to get your shoulders up and back, that is, opening them up outward. *Lengthen and extend your body upward.* Ideally, the palms of your hands should be directly overhead so that your entire body, shoulders included, is in one plane.

Hold for thirty seconds, working your way up to two minutes.

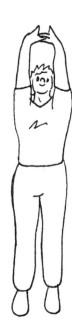

EXERCISES

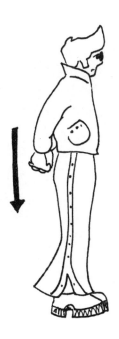

CHEST OPENER

Interlock your fingers behind your back, palms facing upward. Then gently pull downward. Concentrate on allowing your shoulders to roll outward and then down so that you're stretching open the front of your chest. Hold this position for fifteen seconds while trying to get the most lateral portions of your shoulders to open up laterally and downward.

As a variation you can use a railing and simply grab the railing behind you with your palms down. Work on stretching your shoulders down and outward.

FLOOR SIT

Find a comfortable wall. Sit down on the floor with your seat pressed up against the wall. Extend your legs, keeping your legs together and your toes pointing toward the ceiling. You don't have to hold your feet or ankles flexed, but you don't want them rolling out to either side. Relax and gently allow your shoulders and upper back to press back against the wall. Your bottom, the backs of your shoulders, and your head touch the wall. Turn your hands palm up, fingers pointing toward the middle, and place them on your upper thighs. This helps to ensure that your shoulders remain positioned back against the wall. Relax. Are your legs still aligned and your toes still pointing upward? Do you feel the weight evenly distributed on both of your sitting bones? You should feel this exercise in your shoulders, the front of your chest and also often in your groin region and lower back—everywhere.

Hold this position for two to three minutes or longer.

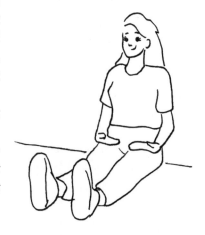

This is also a good exercise to do while watching TV. It properly positions the pelvis and lower back and helps to get the shoulders and upper backs out of the rolled-forward position.

ASTRONAUT

Lie on your back with your bent legs resting on a couch, chair, bed, or ottoman. Take some time to find or make something the correct height—not too high or too low—so that your body can form a ninety-degree angle, and your legs are supported and can rest comfortably on top. Your arms are at your sides, palms up. Make sure your seat is not too far away from whatever you are using. Just relax. Let your pelvis and your lower back relax into the floor. Don't force them or try to make this happen, this is a gravity exercise.

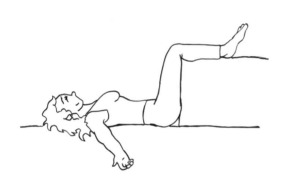

Give this exercise at least five minutes to do its thing. Ten minutes would be even better.

My sister calls this exercise the "Astronaut" because the positioning approximates that of an astronaut in an early space capsule: "Apollo Five, this is Houston . . . can you read me?"

OPENING UP USING EXERCISE BALL, BED, OR BOLSTER

This exercise uses one of those large, colored exercise balls you've probably seen. I highly recommend these balls. There are a great variety of exercises you can do with them to supplement this program. If you don't have a ball, you can use a bed or a large bolster—something you can stretch open over. If you are using the ball, however, simply lie back over the ball and allowing your chest and shoulders to open backwards and downwards toward the floor. Relax and let gravity do its work. By adjusting your hip position on the ball you can work on opening up different

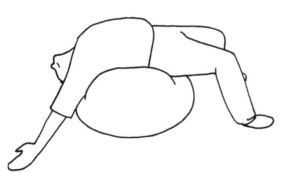

areas of your shoulders, back, and groin. Once you are in position, try moving your arms around, opening up your shoulders further.

Spend around thirty seconds giving your shoulders a deep stretch.

FACE PLANT

This exercise is slightly more challenging but highly recommended. Lie on your stomach with a large firm pillow about eight inches high at arms length above your head. A couch cushion works fine. Extend your legs straight backward and turn your feet inward (pigeon-toed) so that your big toes just touch. Extend your arms palms upward above your head so that they rest on the pillow and are shoulder-width apart. Your face rests on the floor with your nose and chin touching the floor and not tilted up or to either side—hence the name of the exercise. Give this exercise time to work; I know at first it may be very uncomfortable. After a few seconds you should begin to feel this in the backs of your shoulders as they begin to let go and figure out what is going on.

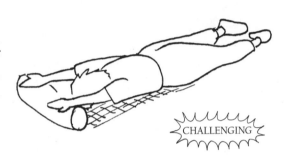

CHALLENGING

Hold for two minutes working up to five minutes.

FACE THE WALL

Stand facing a wall with your feet hip-width apart and your toes turned inward and touching so that you are pigeon-toed. Your chest and nose should be close to the wall. Lift your arms straight above your head and place them on the wall, attempting to place the backs of your hands shoulder-width apart against the wall. At first you may only be able to get the sides of your hands to make contact with the wall.

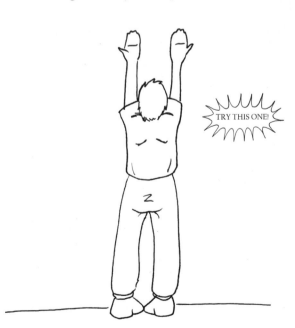

TRY THIS ONE!

Hold this position for one minute, working your way up to three minutes. Focus on keeping your legs and arms straight and your entire body lifted and extending upward. You should feel this in the your shoulders and pelvis.

GLUTE EXERCISES

These exercises strengthen and align the muscles in the buttocks, the backs of the thighs, and the lower back.

BRIDGE LIFT

This is a challenging exercise that also strengthens the back along with the glute muscles. Lie on your back with your knees bent and your feet flat on the floor, hip-width apart, and pointing straight ahead. Your hands should rest comfortably at your sides, palms down. Make sure your body is in a straight line, that is, you don't want to be cocked to one side or the other. Lift your bottom straight up off the floor toward the ceiling. Your weight remains supported by your head, shoulders, arms, and the bottoms of your feet. Lift as high as you can toward the ceiling. Don't just go through the motions; try to get that extra push upward at the top. You should feel this in your buttocks and in your low back. Hold for a second and then lower your bottom slowly back down towards the floor but don't let it touch. When it is an inch or so away, again arch your back and lift up in the air.

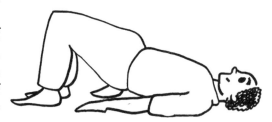

Work up to doing twenty of these. As a variation, you can widen your foot position and also experiment with doing some of your reps with your feet closer or farther away from you.

GLUTE CONTRACTIONS

This is a mild, yet effective exercise that isolates glute activity. Lie on your back with your knees bent and your feet hip-width apart. Now contract only your glute muscles; that is, squeeze together the muscles of your buttocks. Try to isolate and squeeze just the glute muscles and not your thigh or hip muscles. You may put your hands on your bottom to get the feel of doing this properly.

Do twenty contractions.

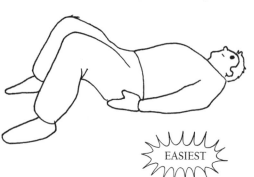

EASIEST

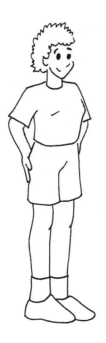

STANDING GLUTE CONTRACTIONS

This is a three-part exercise. Stand with your feet hip-width apart and pointing straight ahead. Contract your buttock muscles in a single, smooth motion, then release.

Do twenty of these. Now turn your feet outward about forty-five degrees and do twenty more. Finally, turn your feet toward the middle so that you are pigeon-toed and do twenty more contractions. These three positions work on slightly different areas of the buttock muscles.

LOCUST LEG LIFTS

Lie on your stomach with your arms at your sides, palms upward. Your chin or forehead is resting on the ground. Keep your head pointing straight ahead; don't lift it while doing this exercise. Your feet are together and pointed straight backward. Now, while keeping your legs straight and pressing down gently with your hands, lift your right leg six to eight inches off the ground and hold it there. *Make sure that both hip bones remain in contact with the ground.* Don't rock or tilt your body in doing this; simply lift your leg straight up toward the ceiling. Keep you toes pointed.

Hold for 15 seconds and then repeat on the other side. Do each side twice.

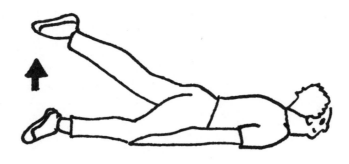

GRAVITY EXERCISES

These exercises place the pelvis and shoulders in an aligned position and allow gravity to do the work.

GROIN STRETCH

This is perhaps the best overall exercise for postural alignment. Its primary effect is to stretch, release, and align the groin muscles. Over time, this exercise will align your hips and allow your shoulders and back to return to a more anatomically correct position.

For this exercise you need something like a chair, a sofa, a bed, an ottoman, or even a coffee table. Take you time and find something the correct height for you. You want something neither too high nor too low so that, when you lie on the floor on your back, one leg can be supported and rest on top of your "platform" forming approximately a ninety-degree angle.

Lie on the floor on your back, bend one leg, and place it on top of whatever you've chosen to use. Stretch the other leg out alongside the object. Make sure your torso is in line with your hips and not cocked to one side. Your bottom should be up close to whatever you are using—almost as if you were sitting in a chair and fell over backward. The toes on the straight leg, that is, the foot alongside the object, should be pointing toward the ceiling, not falling to one side or the other. Use a few pillows or a block of some kind to keep your straight-leg foot from falling out to the side. It is less crucial if your bent leg foot rolls outward slightly. Your arms are at your sides with your palms facing up. Relax. This is a passive exercise where you allow gravity to do the work.

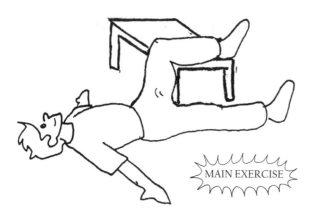

MAIN EXERCISE

Rest in this pose for five minutes, and then switch sides. Make sure you do both sides. It would be even better if you did ten minutes or more on each side.

FLOOR SIT

Find a comfortable wall. Sit down on the floor with your seat pressed up against the wall. Extend your legs, keeping your legs together and your toes pointing toward the ceiling. You don't have to hold your feet or ankles flexed, but you don't want them rolling out to either side. Relax and gently allow your shoulders and upper back to press back against the wall. Your bottom, the backs of your shoulders, and your head touch the wall. Turn your hands palm up, fingers pointing toward the middle, and place them on your upper thighs. This helps to ensure that your shoulders remain positioned back against the wall. Relax. Are your legs still aligned and your toes still pointing upward? Do you feel the weight evenly distributed on both of your sitting bones? You should feel this exercise in your shoulders, the front of your chest and also often in your groin region and lower back—everywhere.

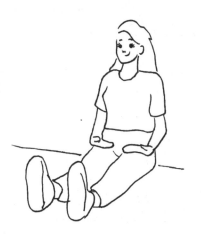

Hold this position for two to three minutes or longer.

This is also a good exercise to do while watching TV. It properly positions the pelvis and lower back and helps to get the shoulders and upper backs out of the rolled-forward position.

ASTRONAUT

Lie on your back with your bent legs resting on a couch, chair, bed, or ottoman. Take some time to find or make something the correct height—not too high or too low—so that your body can form a ninety-degree angle, and your legs are supported and can rest comfortably on top. Your arms are at your sides, palms up. Make sure your seat is not too far away from whatever you are using. Just relax. Let your pelvis and your lower back relax into the floor. Don't force them or try to make this

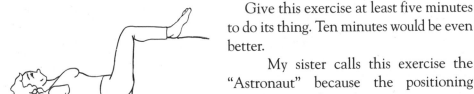

happen, this is a gravity exercise.

Give this exercise at least five minutes to do its thing. Ten minutes would be even better.

My sister calls this exercise the "Astronaut" because the positioning approximates that of an astronaut in an early space capsule: "Apollo Five, this is Houston . . . can you read me?"

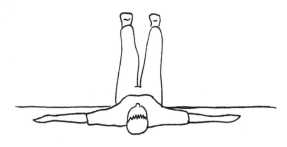

LEGS UP WALL

Lie on the floor, bringing your bottom as close to the wall as possible. The easy way to do this is to sit sideways next to the wall and then turn, sliding your legs up the wall while lying down on your back. Your legs are together, hip-width apart with your toes straight ahead. There is no need to flex or extend the ankles, but don't let your feet roll out to the side. Straighten your legs. If this is impossible, adjust your distance from the wall—moving your seat farther away from the wall makes it easier. Rest your arms at your sides and let your shoulders relax into the floor.

Hold for five minutes or longer. You should feel your back, hips, and shoulders slowly settle into the floor.

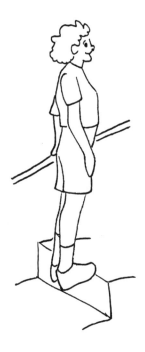

STAIR DROP

Stand with just the balls of your feet (feet pointing straight ahead) on the edge of a stair so that your heels drop downward but don't touch the lower stair. Gently hold onto the railing or wall with one or both hands just to keep your balance. Don't let your pelvis collapse forward or backward, but rather extend and lengthen upward while allowing your heels to drop down. Lift your shoulders up, then back, and down so that you position them properly. As you let your heels relax downward, you should feel a stretch in the back of your calves extending up toward your buttocks.

Hold for two minutes working up to three minutes. Keep a close eye on your alignment. Watch your feet; they will want to turn in or out.

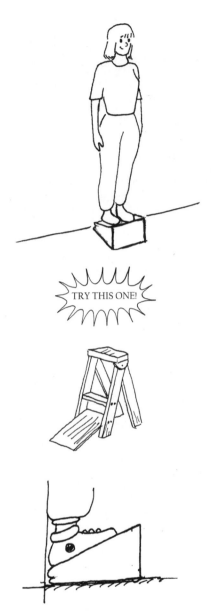

TRY THIS ONE!

SLANT BOARD

A slant board is a simple device that stretches the calf muscles. When used against a wall, it places the body in a aligned position, and is a very powerful tool for postural alignment. However, if you have particularly tight calf muscles, use caution.

You can buy a slant board in some fitness catalogs or you can make one. One alternative is to extend a sturdy piece of wood approximately fifteen inches wide from the bottom rung of short kitchen stepladder. The end of the wood should contact the base of the wall so that it doesn't slide out. By adjusting the distance between the stepladder and the wall, you can adjust the stretch placed on your calves. Six inches of vertical height at the tips of your toes is a good average amount to start with (see the illustrations).

Place the slant board against the wall and stand on it with your back against the wall. Make sure your feet are pointed straight ahead and hip-width apart. Your shoulders and head should be in contact with the wall; your arms are at your sides. This may feel very uncomfortable. As you stay in this position, your body will begin to adjust to this new aligned positioning. Check and readjust your position every once in awhile. Make sure your shoulders and bottom remain in contact with the wall.

Hold this position for at least five minutes; ten minutes would be even better.

EXERCISES

HAMSTRING STRETCHES

These exercises stretch and align the muscles in the backs of the legs.

HAMSTRING STRETCH WITH STRAP

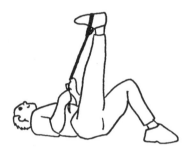

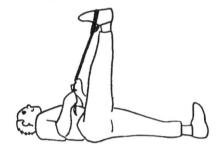

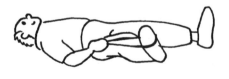

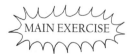

For this exercise you need a belt, towel, or strap—anything readily available will do but a yoga strap works best. Lie on your back with your knees bent and your feet on the floor. Make sure your hips are level; your weight should feel equal on both sides and neither hip should be shifted laterally. Lift your right leg and place the strap around the ball of your foot. Straighten the leg, flexing your toes toward you. Adjust the strap length so that you feel the stretch in your calf muscles and hamstrings. Don't let your hips and shoulders lift off the floor.

Hold for fifteen seconds and then straighten your left leg (the leg without the strap) so that it is now flat on the floor. You may need to adjust the strap again (making it longer) to keep your right leg straight. Hold and stretch for another fifteen seconds. You will feel some of the stretch in your opposite groin; make sure you keep your opposite leg (left) straight as well and don't let it roll out to the side.

Finally, stretch your right leg outward along the floor as high up toward your head as possible. Only stretch as far as you can while keeping your leg straight and maintaining correct alignment. You should feel this in your right groin and a different area of your calf and hamstrings. Stretch for fifteen seconds. Repeat on the other side.

EXERCISES

HAMSTRING STRETCH AT CORNER

No, you're not going to be hanging out on the nearest street corner to do this one. Instead, find a corner wall or doorway in your house. Lie down so that your bottom is close to the wall and one leg extends up the wall while the other leg lies flat on

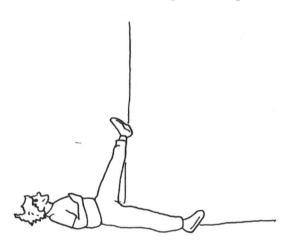

the floor alongside the wall. Work on trying to keep both legs straight while adjusting your distance from the wall to optimize the stretch in your hamstrings. Don't let either foot roll out to the side. You can also flex and extend your feet to gently stretch your calf muscles.

Stretch for thirty seconds and then switch sides.

TRY THIS ONE!

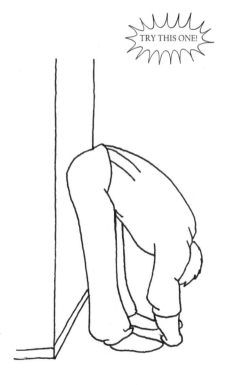

HAMSTRING STRETCH AT WALL

Stand facing outward about ten inches from a wall. Lean back slightly so that only your bottom rests against the wall. Straighten your legs, making sure your feet are hip-width apart and pointing straight ahead. Bend forward at the waist. Keep your back flat and try to avoid hunching it or rounding it forward (see "How to Bend Forward Without Hurting Yourself" Page 109). Grasp your elbows with opposite hands and hang. Relax. While keeping your knees straight, let the weight of your body stretch your lower back and your hamstrings. If this is too difficult, you can place a small block on the floor, reach down, and hold onto that.

Stretch for thirty seconds.

WIDE-LEG FORWARD BEND

Spread your feet so that they are about 3 1/2 to 4 feet apart and pointing straight ahead. Lift your arms, stretching them out to the side— your wrists should be approximately above your ankles. Now, bend forward at the waist keeping your back flat and touch your hands to the floor (see "How to Bend Forward Without Hurting Yourself" Page 109). Your hips should be level—one shouldn't be higher or more forward the other. While keeping your legs straight, adjust your position so that you feel a stretch deep in your hamstrings extending up into your buttocks. If you can't reach anywhere near the floor, place a small block in front of you, reach down, and hold on to that. Be careful and in control. Once you are down, you can move slightly from side to side to stretch tight areas. Moving your bottom backward and upwards accentuates the stretch.

Stretch for thirty seconds.

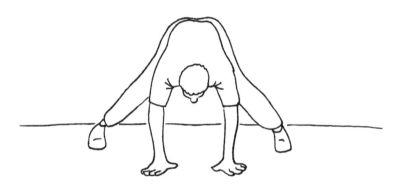

HIP AND GLUTE STRETCHES

These exercises stretch the muscles on the inside and outside of the thighs and buttocks.

HIP STRETCH AT WALL

Lie on your back on the floor several feet from a wall. Place both feet on the wall so that your legs, knees, and hips form ninety-degree angles—just as if you were sitting in a chair. Cross your right foot on top of your left thigh just above the knee.

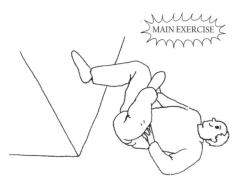

MAIN EXERCISE

Make sure you haven't shifted your hips. Your hips should remain in line; don't let your left leg roll to either side. Press your right thigh outward, opening up deep in the right buttock and groin. You can adjust your distance from the wall, bringing your bottom closer to the wall and making the angles more acute to accentuate the stretch.

Stretch for thirty seconds and then switch sides.

HIP STRETCH ON FLOOR

Lie on your back with your knees bent. Make sure your hips are in line with your torso and that one isn't tilted or out to the side. Cross your right leg so that your right foot rests on your left thigh just above the knee. Stretch the right knee outward, away from your body, while making sure you don't shift or adjust your hips to compensate for the stretch. You should feel this stretch deep in your right buttock.

Stretch for 30 seconds and then switch sides.

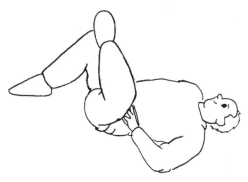

HIP STRETCH ON CHAIR

Sit in a hard-bottomed chair with your back straight and your feet pointing straight ahead hip-width apart. Cross your right leg on top of your left so that your right foot rests on your left thigh just above the knee. Focus on opening your right thigh outward (like opening a book) while stretching your right knee downward. Make sure your hips and back stay aligned so that you maximize the stretch in your right buttock and groin. Usually one side is easier to stretch than the other.

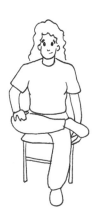

Stretch for thirty seconds and then switch sides.

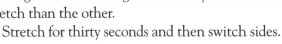

STANDING HIP STRETCH

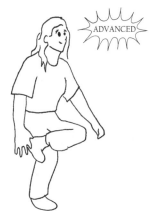

To do this one you have to be able to balance on one foot and have strong knees and thighs. Stand with your feet pointing straight ahead hip-width apart. Squat down slightly and then lift and bring your right foot on top of your left thigh just above the knee. Attempt to open your right thigh outward. Keep your back straight and upright. Accentuate the stretch by squatting farther, bending at the knees, while continuing to open your thigh outward. At first it may be helpful to do this near a wall or something you can hold on to.

Stretch for thirty seconds and then switch sides.

CROSSOVER LEG STRETCH

Lie on your back with your knees bent. Make sure your hips are equally in line with your torso and that one hip isn't tilted or out to the side. Cross your right leg so that your right foot rests on your left thigh just above the knee. Next, twist your hips toward the left so that your right foot comes down toward the floor while remaining in contact with your thigh. Concentrate on pushing your right knee away from your body. You should feel a stretch in your right groin and around your thigh.

Hold and stretch for thirty seconds and then repeat on the opposite side.

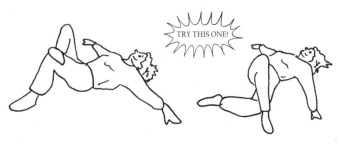

HIP FLEXOR STRETCHES

These exercises stretch and align the muscles in front of the hips.

GROIN STRETCH

This is perhaps the best overall exercise for postural alignment. Its primary effect is to stretch, release, and align the groin muscles. Over time, this exercise will align your hips and allow your shoulders and back to return to a more anatomically correct position.

For this exercise you need something like a chair, a sofa, a bed, an ottoman, or even a coffee table. Take you time and find something the correct height for you. You want something neither too high nor too low so that, when you lie on the floor on your back, one leg can be supported and rest on top of your "platform" forming approximately a ninety-degree angle.

Lie on the floor on your back, bend one leg, and place it on top of whatever you've chosen to use. Stretch the other leg out alongside the object. Make sure your torso is in line with your hips and not cocked to one side. Your bottom should be up close to whatever you are using—almost as if you were sitting in a chair and fell over backward. The toes on the straight leg, that is, the foot alongside the object, should be pointing toward the ceiling, not falling to one side or the other. Use a few pillows or a block of some kind to keep your straight-leg foot from falling out to the side. It is less crucial if your bent leg foot rolls outward slightly. Your arms are at your sides with your palms facing up. Relax. This is a passive exercise where you allow gravity to do the work.

Rest in this pose for five minutes, and then switch sides. Make sure you do both sides. It would be even better if you did ten minutes or more on each side.

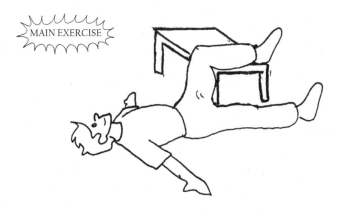

MAIN EXERCISE

LUNGE

Step forward with your right leg, bending your knee so that your body comes down close to the top of your right thigh. Your right foot should be pointing straight ahead with your ankle in front of or directly below but not behind your knee. Your back leg remains straight. You may either lay your left foot out flat on the floor behind you (toes pointing back, not out to either side) or remain on your toes with your foot straight. If you are able to, gently rest your hands on the floor on either side of your leg trying to keep your body close to upright. Otherwise do this exercise next to a couch or similar object and use your hands to steady yourself. To accentuate the stretch focus on slightly lowering your left hip toward the floor while keeping your left knee straight and lifting it. Watch your alignment.

Stretch for fifteen to thirty seconds then repeat on the opposite side.

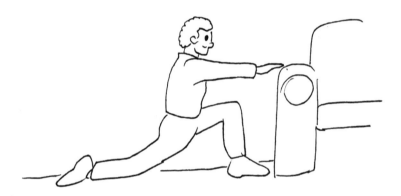

LEG TO CHEST

Lie on your back in an aligned position. Bend your right leg and bring it to your chest, wrapping your fingers around your leg several inches below your knee or around your ankle. It helps if you bring your knee slightly outward first before bringing it in and toward your chest. Pull down firmly with your hands to bring your knee as close to your chest as possible. Your head remains flat on the floor. Keep your back flat against the ground—don't let it arch. You should feel a stretch in both groin regions and in your right buttock. Make sure you try to keep your outstretched leg straight (not rolled out to the side), your toes pointing toward the ceiling, and the entire back of your thigh and calf in contact with the floor. Give this one time to work.

Hold and stretch for thirty seconds and then repeat on the opposite side.

For a deeper stretch, you can do this exercise while lying on a table. Your buttocks should be near the edge of the table and your straight leg hanging off the table (don't let it roll to the side). Keep your back flat against the table—don't let it arch. Again, pull your bent leg toward your chest. Watch your alignment.

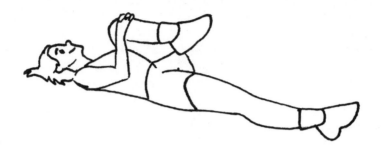

SINGLE-LEGGED TABLE STRETCH

Stand facing a table. Lift your right leg and place it on top of the table directly in front of you. Use your hands to gently hold onto the table top. Adjust your position so that the groin of your standing leg is touching the edge of the table. Your standing foot remains pointing straight ahead.

Work on getting your right leg to lie flat on the table at a ninety-degree angle to your body without letting it roll to either side. Your toes should point toward the ceiling. *Lift and extend upward* so that you are standing straight with neither too much nor too little arch in your back. You should feel a stretching in your right groin. Make sure your hips haven't rocked to either side.

Hold for one minute and then repeat with the opposite leg.

Once you have mastered the basic pose, you can try gently bending forward for a few seconds and reaching toward your toes. Make sure you keep your back flat and don't bend your knees when you bend forward.

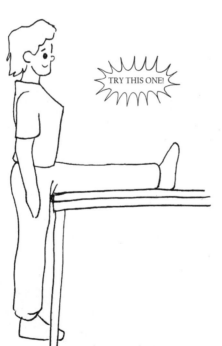

TRY THIS ONE!

HIP OPENERS

These exercises stretch and align the muscles in the pelvis and hips that allow us to rotate our legs outward.

FROG

Lie on your back. Bring your feet together so that the bottoms of your feet touch. Allow your knees to fall out to the side. Make sure your weight is evenly centered on both 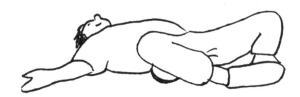 sitting bones. The closer your feet are to your body the deeper the stretch; the farther away, the easier. If this is terribly uncomfortable on your knees, you can place pillows or a folded blanket under your knees to give them some support. You should feel the stretch deep in your groins. Try to relax and slightly rotate your thighs outward to deepen the stretch.

Hold for one minute.

Feet closer to you = HARDER.

Feet farther away = EASIER.

FROG AT WALL

This is a variation of the basic frog exercise. Lie on the floor with your bottom as close to the wall as possible. The easy way to do this is to sit sideways next to the wall and then turn while lying down on your back so that your feet slide up the

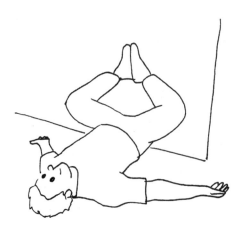

wall. Bring the soles of your feet together and allow your knees to open up out to the sides. Adjust your position to deepen the stretch by bringing your bottom closer to the wall if it has slid away. Make sure your weight remains evenly centered on both hips. Feet closer toward you equals a deeper stretch, while feet higher up the wall makes it slightly easier.

Hold and stretch for one minute.

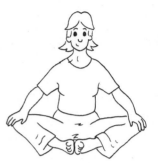

COBBLER POSE

Sit with your back against the wall. Place the soles of your feet together, allowing your knees to fall out to the side. Rest your hands on your thighs and gently press your knees downward. Make sure you keep your back straight against the wall and are not hunched forward.

Hold for one minute. You can do the same exercise without the wall, but you need to remain vigilant in keeping your back upright without the assistance of the wall.

SIDE-SITTING

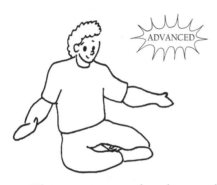

Sit on the floor with your knees bent and your legs lying on the floor to the right side. Your right foot points outward and your left foot touches your right thigh. Trying to keep your back vertical, you shoulders level, and both of your sitting bones touching the floor. You should feel this stretch in your right outer hip and back.

Hold for up to three minutes and then switch sides.

This exercise stretches the muscles on the outside of the hips and back, demanding your hips to open up equally on both sides. You'll probably find that one side is markedly tighter than the other. If this exercise hurts your knees, don't do it.

REVERSE FROG AT WALL

In this exercise the frog is on his belly. Lie on the floor on your stomach close to a wall with your knees bent at about ninety degrees. Spread each knee outward while keeping your toes touching. Adjust your position so that your feet slide up the wall

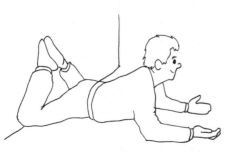

and your knees are close to the base of the wall. Make sure the weight is evenly balanced on both hips. Lift up slightly, supporting your weight on your forearms and palms, which extend straight ahead. You should feel a stretch in your back and both groins. Adjust your position so that the stretch is right for you.

Work your way up to holding and stretching in this position for three minutes.

INNER THIGH STRENGTHENERS

These exercises strengthen and align the muscles on the inside of the legs.

PILLOW SQUEEZES ON FLOOR

Lie on your back with your knees bent and feet hip-width apart. Make sure your weight is evenly distributed on both hips and that one isn't cocked out to the side. Place a small pillow or cushion between your knees. Your hands are at your sides, palms up. Squeeze the pillow between your knees and release. Use the muscles on the inside of your thighs to do the squeezes.

Work up to forty squeezes.

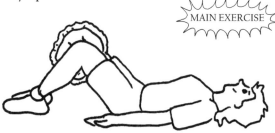

PILLOW SQUEEZES ON CHAIR

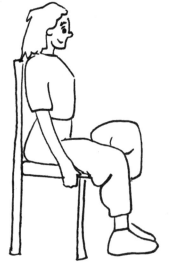

Sit upright in a hard-bottomed chair with your feet pointing straight ahead and hip-width apart. Place a small pillow or cushion between your knees. Your hands are in your lap, palms up; this helps keep your shoulders back. With your back remaining straight, gently squeeze the pillow between your knees. Hold for a few seconds, then release.

Work up to forty squeezes.

EXERCISES

BIG BALL SQUEEZES

Straddle a large exercise ball with your thighs so that the ball is off the ground and held between your thighs. Point your feet straight ahead if possible. With your knees slightly bent, squeeze and release the ball between your thighs and legs.

Work up to forty squeezes.

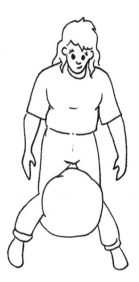

CROSSED LEG LIFT

Lie on the floor on your right side with either your head resting on your outstretched right arm or your elbow bent and supporting your head in your hand. Make sure your body is in a straight line and not cocked to one side or the other. Bend your left leg and place your left foot behind your right knee. Recheck your alignment. Now, lift your right (bottom) leg up toward the ceiling, hold for a second, and then release back down. Keep the leg you are lifting straight.

Work up to forty lifts. Repeat on the other side.

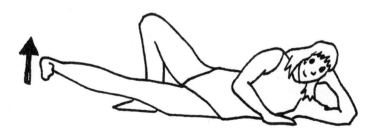

LOWER EXTREMITY STRENGTHENERS

These exercises strengthen and align the major weight-bearing muscles in the legs and back.

SITTING AND STANDING

This is what we do all day. Sit down and stand up. Stand up and sit down. So let's build our strength and alignment by doing it right. Don't be deceived. This is harder than it looks to do properly. Find a chair with a hard bottom, not a cushy office chair or couch. Sit down. You want your weight evenly distributed on both of your sitting bones, a slight curve in your lower back, and a slight lift to your chest. Shoulders are pulled gently back and down. Hands rest at your sides. Your feet are hip-width apart and your toes point straight ahead. Stand straight up. No pushing on your thighs or helping with your hands. No leaning forward or off to one side. Imagine a string attached to the top of your head pulling you gently upward. Try to avoid the corkscrew effect of writhing your way upward. Make sure you become fully erect and take a moment to bring your shoulders all the way back. Now, sit back down in the same controlled manner.

Repeat twenty of these. Do only as many as you can while maintaining correct alignment. Often our leg muscles have gotten weak and we have a tendency to want to cheat by using our back or side muscles or our hands to push off. Once you start compensating, quit. If it is too hard to do any of these, use a higher chair or sit on the edge of the chair, or put some big pillows on a chair to give you an extra boost.

This is also a good exercise to incorporate into your day; anytime you get up, try to get up without using your hands to push off.

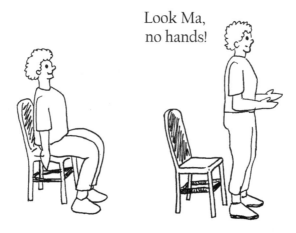

Look Ma, no hands!

LEG LIFTS

This is a milder exercise that isolates and works the muscles that flex your hips. Lie on your back with your knees bent and your feet a comfortable distance from your body. Your arms rest at your sides. Lift your right foot four inches off the ground and then lower it back down. Let the muscle deep in your groin do the work and don't use your hands to push into the ground.

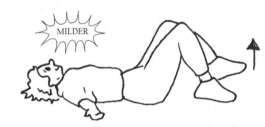

Do twenty of these and then switch sides. Work up to doing forty. When you can do forty you can easily progress to one of the other exercises.

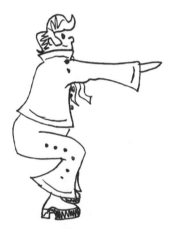

IMAGINARY CHAIR

Stand with your feet hip-width apart and your toes pointing straight ahead. Extend your arms out in front of you at shoulder level with your palms down. Now slowly lower yourself down, bending your knees and using your thigh muscles as if you were sitting down on an imaginary chair. Keep your back straight—try not to bend forward and try to keep your weight toward your heels. The lower you go, the more demanding it is on your thigh muscles. Challenge yourself without compromising your form or alignment.

Hold for fifteen seconds; over time, work up to a full minute. Then rest for a few seconds and repeat, holding the pose for half as long as you did the first time.

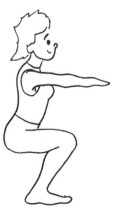

SQUATS

Stand with your feet pointing straight ahead and hip-width apart. Extend your arms out in front of you. While keeping your back straight and your shoulders back, bend your knees and squat down toward the floor. Don't let your knees flare out to one side or the other; try to keep them pointing straight ahead as you bend down. Bend down as far as you comfortably can and then lift back up. If this exercise hurts your knees, don't bend down so far.

Do twenty of these. Over time work at bending lower and lower.

WALL BENCH

Find a comfortable wall. Stand with your back toward the wall and your feet pointing straight ahead and hip-width apart. Lean back against the wall. Slide your back down the wall and your feet forward so that you are sitting in the air with your lower back and shoulders pressed into the wall. Your knees should be slightly behind or above your ankles forming approximately a ninety-degree angle, but they should not be forward of your ankles. If this is too painful on your knees, slide up the wall a little.

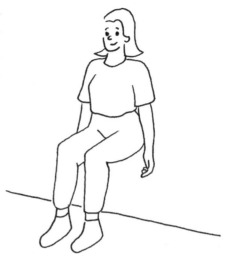

Your goal is to work your way up to holding this position for two minutes. At first fifteen seconds may be enough.

REACHING DOWN UNDER

No, this has nothing to do with Australia. What we're doing here is mimicking the movement of reaching out one hand to pick up a fallen object under a table.

Stand five or six feet away from a table with your feet together. Imagine an object has fallen just under the edge of the table. Step forward on one leg, bend, and pretend to grab the object. Try to keep your body in line and not swinging out to one side or the other. Once you have touched the spot where the object was, return to your starting position with your feet together.

Do ten of these, stepping forward with the right leg; then do ten using the other leg. Work your way up until you can do twenty on each side.

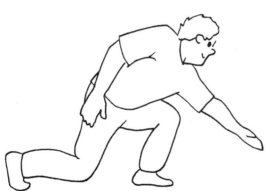

It may be difficult to do even one to begin with. The front of your thigh may quiver; your buttock muscles may feel tight; you may feel as if your knees are going to give way. Welcome to the club. Do the best you can while maintaining somewhat decent alignment.

PICK-UPS

Ugh! Another exercise where we have to bend down. We're hammering away at the leg muscles because that's where so many of us are weak. Or else we're clumsy and keep dropping things. In any case, imagine that there are twenty objects on the floor directly in front of you. Stand with feet hip-width apart and pointing straight ahead. Bend your knees, crouch down, and pretend to pick up the first object. Make sure your knees bend straight ahead. We all have a favorite side; avoid splaying your knees out to one side or the other or leading with one foot. Make sure you go far enough down so that you can touch the floor. Now stand back up. Once you are all the way up, take a second to move your shoulders back—don't leave them rolled forward. Then crouch down again. You get the idea.

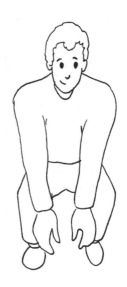

Once you've picked up all twenty objects you can stop.

GETTING DOWN AND GETTING UP

They say it's not the falling down in our lives that matters, but it's the getting up afterward. This exercise helps that. Sit down on the floor with your legs bent out to the right side. Your weight should be on both hips and your back should be straight. Now stand up. Oh, one more thing—no using your hands to push off. Keep your hands somewhere in the air like a bird. Once you are standing, sit back down on the floor, this time letting your legs bend to the opposite side, the left side. Again, no using your hands to ease yourself down. Once you are settled completely down, get up again.

Do twenty of these— ten to each side.

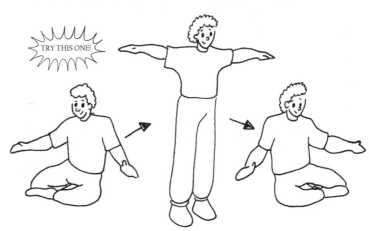

TRY THIS ONE!

OUTER THIGH STRENGTHENERS

These exercises strengthen the muscles on the outside of the thighs.

STANDING SIDE LEG LIFTS

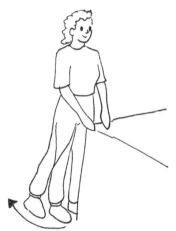

Stand sideways several feet from a counter or similar object. Hold on to the counter with your inside hand. Your feet should be pointing straight ahead and hip-width apart. Lift your outside leg laterally, as high as you comfortably can while keeping both your body and your leg straight. The foot on the lifted leg remains pointing straight ahead. Try to stay vertical while doing this exercise. Avoid leaning or bending to the side but, rather, make sure you let the muscles on the sides of your thighs do the work. When you start having to lean, it's time to quit.

Do twenty of these or until you begin to have to alter your alignment. Repeat on the opposite side.

SIDE-LYING LEG LIFTS

Lie on the right side of your body. Your right elbow is bent with your hand supporting your head. Make sure your body is in one plane (or as close as possible). You don't want your bottom sticking out backward, or your body to be tilted in either direction. Lift your uppermost leg straight toward the ceiling, as high as you comfortably can without altering your alignment. Your toes remain pointed in the same direction as the front of your body.

Do twenty of these or until you begin to alter your alignment. Repeat on the opposite side.

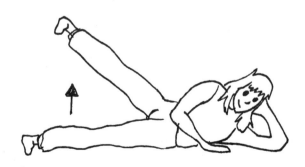

PELVIC RANGE-OF-MOTION EXERCISES

These exercises encourage increased movement in the pelvis and lower back.

CATS AND DOGS

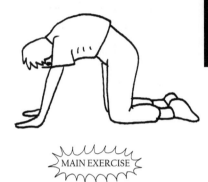

MAIN EXERCISE

Get down on your hands and knees so that your back forms a small table. Your hands should be directly below your shoulders with your fingers pointing forward. Your knees should be directly below your hips, forming a right angle. Now, exhale and arch your back upward like a cat. Do this slowly and consciously making sure you focus on curving your neck (chin toward chest), your upper back, your lower back, and your pelvis so that you form one smooth curve with the back of your body. Do not strain, but make sure you stretch as far as you can. *Focus particularly on getting the last few degrees of tilt to your pelvis.*

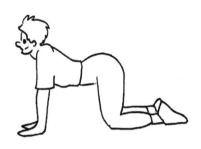

Hold for a few seconds then slowly arch in the other direction. While keeping your hands and knees where they are, arch your head and neck upward, your upper and lower back downward, and lift your buttocks into the air opening them outward. Again, try to make sure you get the last few degrees of tilt to your pelvis so that you feel it in your groins. This is the dog stretch.

Hold for a few seconds and then smoothly transition to the cat stretch. Repeat ten cycles.

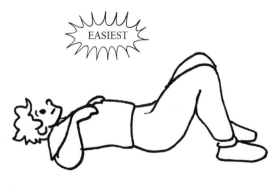

EASIEST

PELVIC TILTS

Lie on your back with your knees bent and your arms comfortably at your sides, palms up. Your hips are centered and your feet are hip-width apart. Gently contract your abdominal muscles, bringing the small of your back flat onto the floor or as close as you can. You should feel a tightening

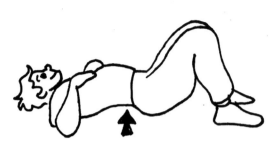

in your abdomen as your pelvis tilts backward toward the floor. Hold for a few seconds, then arch your back in the opposite direction and hold for a few seconds. Initiate the movement by tilting your pelvis, and make sure you maximize your movement in both directions.

Repeat twenty of these.

STANDING CATS AND DOGS

In this exercise our cats and dogs have somehow assumed a two-legged position, perhaps attempting to become human. Stand with your feet hip-width apart and facing forward. Put your hands on your thighs just above your knees so that you are leaning halfway forward. Arch your neck, entire back, and pelvis upward in one smooth motion, letting your head drop slightly downward with your chin coming

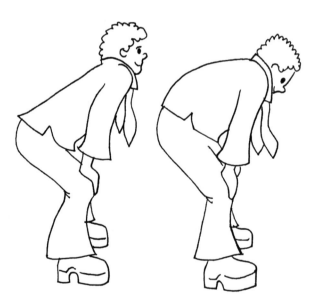

toward your chest. *Make sure you get the last few degrees of tilt from your pelvis.*

Hold for a few seconds then transition through your starting position into the standing dog stretch. Your back becomes concave and your head and upper chest curve upward while your pelvis tilts downward. Your hands stay on your knees throughout.

Hold for a few seconds. Repeat ten cycles.

DOWNWARD DOG

This is a classic yoga exercise. Some yoga teachers say that if you do only one yoga exercise, this is the one to do. It stretches out the entire back of the body including the lower back and hamstrings. Get on the floor on your hands and knees. Your hands are directly under your shoulders, your knees are hip-width apart. Now, while leaving your hands and feet where they are, slowly push yourself up, lifting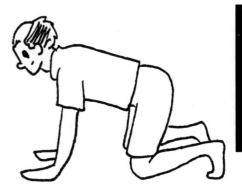

your bottom high in the air so that your body forms a triangle. Your hands are evenly spaced with your fingers pointing forward; your feet are hip-width apart with your toes pointing forward. Your back should be straight, that is, not sagging toward the floor nor overly lifting or arching upward. This can be difficult if you aren't used to it. Ideally, you want your weight evenly balanced between your hands and feet. If you can get your heels to the ground, that's great; if not, don't worry about it but keep your feet pointing straight ahead. Focus on lifting your rear end *up* and *back*.

Hold for fifteen to thirty seconds.

Alternative: If you can't do the whole pose, that's okay. Instead, just get down on your hands and knees (with feet and hands pointing straight ahead) and push up in any manner so that your weight is on your hands and feet. Don't worry initially about how straight things your back is. Just get the feel of supporting yourself on your hands and feet.

Doing this even for a few seconds begins to strengthen muscles and provides a needed stretch to the back of your body.

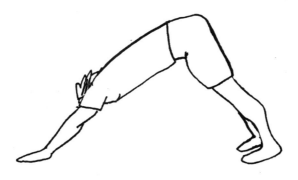

QUADRICEPS STRETCHES

These exercises stretch the large muscles in the front of the thighs.

STANDING QUAD STRETCH

Stand facing a counter, a wall, or the back of a chair—something you can hold on to. Hold on with your left hand and bend your right leg behind you. Grab the top of your foot with your right hand pulling your right foot toward your right buttock. Keep your thighs parallel. Don't allow your bent leg to splay out to the side. Keep your back lifted and straight; holding on to the chair or counter helps you maintain this alignment. If you hunch forward or backward or tilt your pelvis, you won't maximize the stretch in your thigh where you want it. If done properly, you should feel this stretch across the entire front of your thigh and into the groin.

Hold and stretch for thirty seconds and then repeat on the opposite side.

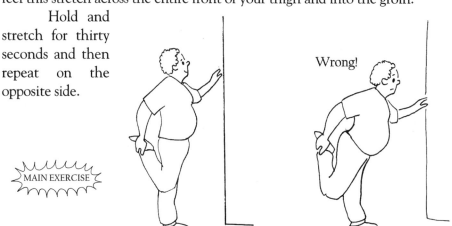

MAIN EXERCISE

Wrong!

SIDE-LYING QUAD STRETCH

Lie on your right side with your legs straight. Reach behind you with your left hand and grab the top of your left foot. Push your left thigh backward while pulling on your foot to feel a deep stretch in your thigh and left groin. Your left thigh is parallel to or behind your right thigh. If you stick your bottom too far back, you won't be maximizing the stretch in the front of the thigh where you want it. If you arch

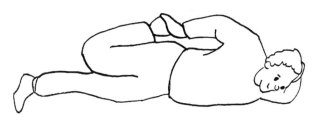

your back too much, your lumbar region will be taking the stretch rather than the thigh.

Hold and stretch for thirty seconds and then repeat on the opposite side.

JAPANESE SITTING POSE

This sitting pose helps align the spine while stretching the hips and quadriceps muscles. There is a great amount of variation in people's ability to do this, so you have to be willing to adjust the position (as will be explained) to find a variation that works for you.

Sit down on the floor Japanese style with your legs bent underneath you so that you are sitting on your heels and your thighs are together with your knees pointing straight ahead. It is important that your toes point straight back or toward the middle and are not flared open to the sides, which puts a strain on the knees. You should feel the stretch in the tops of your thighs. Keep your upper body vertical; don't lean.

Sit for two minutes.

If this terribly painful to the tops of your feet, put some padding under your feet or place a small cushion or folded blanket under your bottom to ease some of the pressure on them. It also helps to grab the tops of both calf muscles from behind just below your knees and pull them down and to the sides to take some of the strain off your knees.

Once you have mastered the basic pose without using any props, you can start to lean backward. Place your hands behind you and start to lean backward. With time, you may be able to settle back on your elbows or even all the way down on your back. Be careful. If this is too painful on your knees, go back to the basic pose. The important thing is to find a variation of this exercise that stretches the front of your thighs for you. Listen to your body and don't overdo.

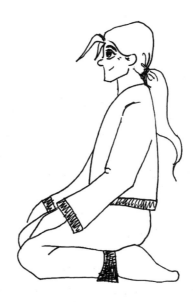

SHOULDER RANGE-OF-MOTION EXERCISES

These exercise help to restore strength and range of motion to the shoulders and upper back.

ARM CIRCLES

Stand with your feet hip-width apart. Lift your arms out to the sides, shoulder high. Relax your shoulders so that they are not hunched up around your neck. Your arms should be straight and level.

   With your thumbs pointing forward make thirty small circles (ten inches in diameter) in the forward direction. Then point your thumbs backward and your palms up and do thirty circles in the reverse direction. Strive to open up your chest and push your shoulders back without letting them rise up around your ears.

   Once you get used to doing the small circles, try doing a set maximizing the rotation of your arms. Everything else remains the same except on the forward circles tilt your hands so that they are facing backwards (the backs of your hands face forward) and you feel the stretch in a different area of your shoulders. For the backward circles, exaggerate the tilt of your hands backward.

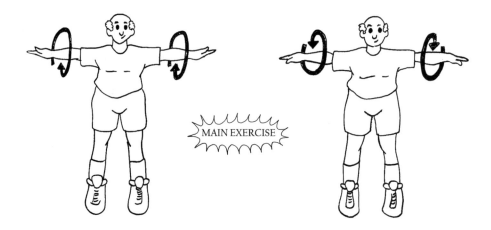

MAIN EXERCISE

SITTING ARM CIRCLES

Sit in a firm, hard-bottomed chair with your feet pointing straight ahead and hip-width apart. Extend your spine, that is, sit up as straight as possible. Lift your arms so that they are shoulder level and out to the sides.

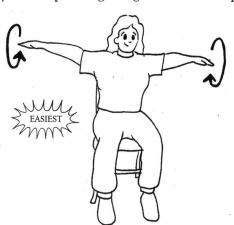

Keeping your arms straight and with your thumbs pointing straight ahead, make thirty small circles (ten inches in diameter) in the forward direction. Now turn your hands so that your palms are up and your thumbs are pointing toward the back. Make thirty small circles in the reverse direction.

EASIEST

ELBOW CURLS

Stand with your feet hip-width apart and pointing straight ahead. Bend your elbows and touch the tips of your fingers to your temples just above your ears. Your elbows should be splayed out like wings. Open them up as wide as you can while keeping your fingers in contact with your temples. Now move both elbows forward—keeping your fingers in contact with your temples—while trying to get your elbows to meet in front of your face. *Stretch* to make your elbows meet. Then pull your elbows back again. remembering to allow them to go as far back as possible, again, while keeping your fingers in contact with your temples.

That's one. Do twenty of these.

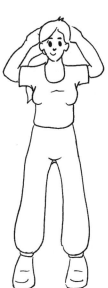

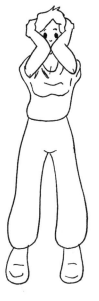

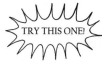

TRY THIS ONE!

ANGEL ARMS AT THE WALL

Stand with your back to the wall. Start with your palms facing outward at your sides. Slowly move your arms above your head until your fingers touch. Work toward keeping your hands, elbows, and shoulders in contact with the wall at all times.

Do ten of these.

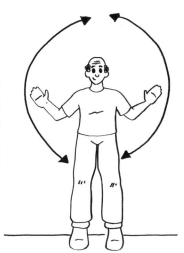

ANGEL ARMS ON CHAIR

Place a hard-bottomed chair with a narrow back against a wall so that you are sitting facing away from the wall. Start with your palms facing outward at your sides in contact with the wall, then slowly move your arms above your head keeping contact with the wall until your fingers touch. Work toward keeping your hands, elbows, and shoulders in contact with the wall at all times.

Do ten of these.

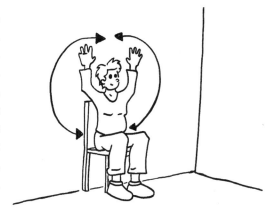

ANGEL ARMS

Remember when you were a kid and made snow angels. Lie on your back with your knees bent and your feet hip-width apart. Start with your arms at your sides on the floor, palms up. While keeping your arms in contact with the floor, slowly slide your

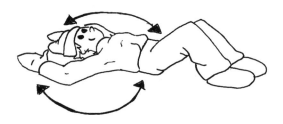

hands up above your head bending your arms slightly at the elbows until your thumbs meet above your head.

Repeat ten times. Try to keep your shoulders in continual contact with the ground.

BREASTSTROKE

No, you don't need to get into the water. Stand with your feet hip-width apart and facing forward. Bring your hands together in front of your chest in a "prayer" position with your elbows pointing out to the sides. Then move your hands directly upward until they are above your head. Try to keep your shoulders pulled back. Now turn your hands palm out and sweep your outstretched arms through the air down to your sides and then back up into prayer position. Do this in one continuous motion. Be precise and controlled in your movements.

Do ten. You're swimming!

Now you need to swim in the opposite direction. Start with your hands palms together above your head. Remember, try to keep your shoulders back. Bring your hands straight down into prayer position then continue down, sweeping them out to the sides, palms up. Finally, bring them back up above your head in one continual motion.

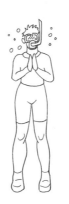 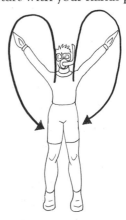

Do ten. You're swimming—backwards!

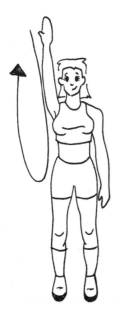

BACKSTROKE

Stand with your hands at your sides. Swing one arm at a time forward and then up and over your head and back around making a big sideways circle with your arm. Keep your arm as close to your body and your head as possible, and try to avoid swaying or twisting. Focus on accessing those areas of your shoulders that don't usually get a stretch.

Then go in the reverse direction. Swing one arm at a time backward and then up and around again, trying to keep your arm close to your body and head.

Do five of each with each arm.

For both of these exercises, altering your hand position (turned inward, turned outward) during some of the circles can stretch different areas of your shoulders.

SHOULDER AND UPPER BACK STRENGTHENERS

These exercises strengthen the muscles surrounding the shoulders, between the shoulders blades, and in the upper back.

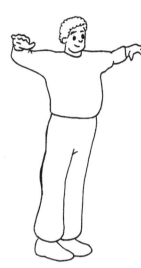

STANDING SHOULDER SQUEEZES

Stand with your feet pointing straight ahead and hip-width apart. Lift your arms up to the sides so that they are even with your shoulders. Bend your elbows so that they form ninety-degree angles to the front. Now move your elbows backward gently contracting and squeezing the muscles between your shoulder blades together. You want to feel the muscles between your shoulder blades contracting and doing the work; don't just push your elbows backward.

Do twenty of these.

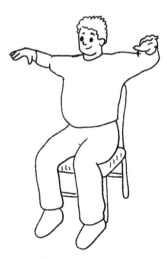

SITTING SHOULDER SQUEEZES

Sit on a hard-bottomed chair, making sure your weight is evenly distributed on both sitting bones and your feet are pointing straight ahead. With your bent elbows out to your sides at shoulder height, move your elbows backward while gently squeezing your shoulder blades together.

Do twenty.

AIRPLANE

Lie on your stomach with your legs stretched out and your feet pigeon-toed so that your big toes touch. Extend your arms out to the sides at shoulder level with your palms facing downward. Now, in one controlled movement, lift your head, shoulders, upper back, and arms off the floor. Try to initiate the movement from your tailbone region. Once you are up, focus on lifting your arms in an up and backward direction. You are now cleared for take-off.

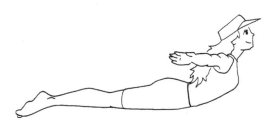

Hold for fifteen to thirty seconds or longer, rest for a few seconds and repeat. At first, you may try locking your feet underneath a couch or similar object for added support.

PUSHUPS

Push-ups are an all-around strengthening exercise. They strengthen our shoulder, chest, upper back, and arm muscles as well as help build core strength. Here are three variations. Do the one that matches your present strength level, and then over time, as you improve try a harder version.

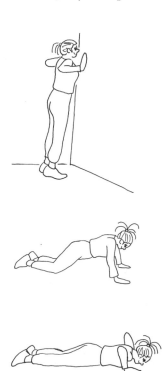

1. For the easiest (mildest) version, stand facing a corner of room about three feet away from the wall. Place one hand on each wall at shoulder height. Let yourself relax toward the wall while bending your elbows. You should feel this between your shoulder blades. Then push yourself back upright so that your arms are straight. Do ten.

2. Get down on the floor for a traditional pushup, except keep your knees on the floor. Place your hands on the floor with your fingers pointing straight ahead just in front of your shoulders. Use your arm, shoulder, and chest muscles to push up.

Work up to ten and then to twenty. Stop once your form begins to falter (compensation).

3. This is the traditional pushup. Make sure your back is straight and that your bottom is neither sagging toward the floor nor lifting high in the air. Work on doing only a few with correct form and then work your way up to doing ten and then to twenty.

SHOULDER SQUEEZES AND OVERHEADS ON FLOOR

This is a two-part exercise.

1. Lie on your back with your knees bent. Bend your elbows and place them in line with your shoulders. Press your elbows into the ground while equally contracting the area between your shoulder blades. You want to feel the muscles between your shoulder blades contract. Do twenty of these.

2. Next, grasp your hands together and lift them above your head. Attempt to press your clenched hands into the floor above your head. Try to keep your elbows straight and your back from arching. If you can't reach the floor with your hands, you can put a pillow or cushion there and press into that. This is both a strength-

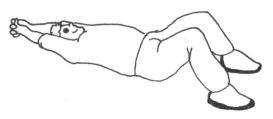

ening and range-of motion-exercise. Come back to your starting position and repeat this ten to twenty times making sure you press downward for a few seconds each time. You should feel this in your shoulders and between your shoulder blades.

SHOULDER SQUEEZES AND OVERHEADS IN ASTRONAUT POSE

Lie on your back with your legs bent at a ninety-degree angle and resting on top of a chair, block, or ottoman. Make sure your hips are in line and your seat is close to the base of the chair.

1. Bend your elbows and place them in line with your shoulders. Press your elbows into the ground while contracting the area between your shoulder blades. Do twenty of these.

2. Now, grasp your hands together and lift them above your head. Attempt to press your clenched hands into the floor above your head. Try to keep your elbows straight. If you can't reach the floor with your hands, you can put a pillow or cushion there and press into that. Come back to your starting position and repeat this

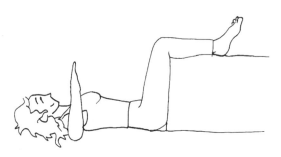

ten to twenty times, making sure you press downward into the floor above your head for a few seconds each time. You should feel this in your shoulders and between your shoulder blades.

SHOULDER SQUEEZES AND OVERHEADS ON CHAIR WITH BACK AGAINST WALL

This is a two-part exercise.

1. Place a hard-bottomed chair with a narrow back against a wall so that you are sitting facing away from the wall. Bend your elbows and place them in line with your shoulders. Press your elbows against the wall while contracting the area between your shoulder blades. You want to feel the muscles between your shoulder blades contract. Do twenty of these.

2. Next, grasp your hands together and lift them above your head. Attempt to press your clenched hands against the wall above your head. Try to keep your elbows straight and your back from arching. If you can't reach the wall above you with your hands, simply go as far as you can while trying to feel a stretch in your shoulders. *Avoid over-arching your back.*

Come back to your starting position and repeat this ten to twenty times of these making sure you press your hands backward toward the wall for a few seconds each time.

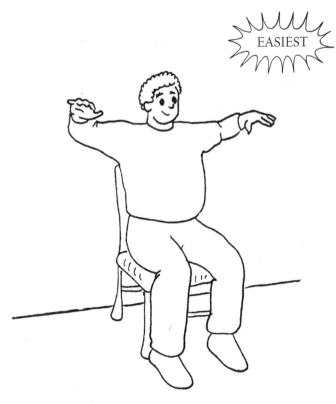

EASIEST

SIDE STRETCHES

These exercises primarily stretch and strengthen the muscles along the sides of the body.

TRIANGLE

This is a classic yoga pose. Stand with your feet about three and one half feet apart and your toes pointing straight ahead. Lift your arms to shoulder level. Your wrists should be approximately above your ankles. Turn your right foot out ninety degrees

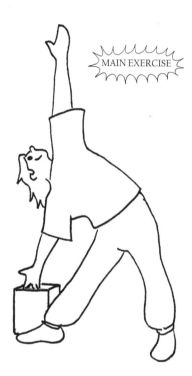

MAIN EXERCISE

and your left foot in forty-five degrees. The heel of your right foot should line up with the arch of your left foot. Bend sideways at the waist bringing your right hand down toward your right ankle. If you can, touch your fingers to the floor at the outside of your foot. Otherwise, grab onto your right ankle or calf as far down as you can go. Another alternative is to place a small block to the outside of your foot and hold onto that. Keep your legs straight and only bend as far as you can while maintaining straight legs. Your left arm lifts above your head, pointing straight toward the ceiling. You can turn your head and look toward your left hand or simply look straight ahead. *Focus on opening your topmost hip up and outward rather than collapsing or bending forward.*

Hold for fifteen to thirty seconds, then come up slowly and repeat on the opposite side.

TRIANGLE AT THE WALL

Stand with your back to the wall. Spread your legs three and one half feet apart. Turn your right foot out ninety degrees and your left foot in forty-five degrees. Your left heel should be close to the wall and right foot a few inches away. Bend toward the right, keeping your pelvis and back against the wall as much as possible. Grab your ankle or as far down as you can while keeping both legs straight. The key to this exercise is not to bend forward but, rather, to bend to the side, keeping your

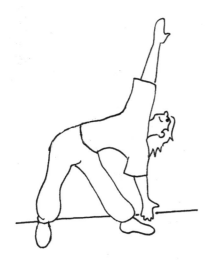

body in the same plane as the wall. Lift your left arm up so that the back of your hand touches the wall. Turn your head and look up toward your left hand if you can. Adjust your position to maximize the stretch along the sides of your body.

Hold for fifteen to thirty seconds, then come up slowly and repeat on the opposite side.

THE CLOCK

Stand with your feet three and one half feet apart. Lift both arms above your head, keeping your palms facing forward and interlocking your thumbs. This is twelve o'clock. Now slowly rotate your torso and arms to the right, keeping them as close to the same plane as your body as you can. Don't fold forward. Try to keep your shoulders opening outward. Pretend your arms are the hands on a clock. Proceed slowly around the clock until you are hanging completely downward at six o'clock. Relax for a few seconds and then continue around until once again your arms are pointing upward at twelve o'clock. Do this exercise slowly and in control. You should feel this in your flanks and on the sides of your body.

Go around the clock three times in the forward direction and then three times in reverse. Then it's time to quit.

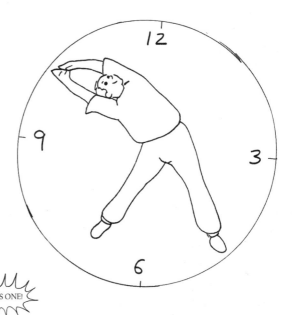

TRY THIS ONE!

TWISTS

These exercises encourage symmetrical full range of motion of the hips and shoulders.

FLOOR TWIST

Lie on the floor on your right side with your knees forming a ninety-degree angle. Your arms are out to the right, one on top of the other in line with your shoulders. While leaving your knees in place, slowly rotate your upper (left) arm and shoulder upward and across to your left side. You should feel this in your left hip and shoulder. The idea is to, over time, get your left shoulder and arm to lie flat on the floor while keeping your knees in position. Go slow and be gentle with this—listen to your body. You may also gently press down on your right knee with your right hand to accentuate the stretch. Over time, attempt to turn your head so that it looks away from the bent knee side.

Hold for one minute. Repeat on the other side.

Bringing your knees up tighter and higher (closer to your arms) makes this exercise more demanding. Stretching out your knees slightly and bringing them downward toward your feet makes it easier. Adjust the position so you feel a stretch appropriate to your level of flexibility.

Make sure that your body remains symmetrically aligned. Even though your hips are twisting, they should not be jutted out to the side. Your arms should remain level with your shoulders on both sides. When you are in the full position, focus on extending and lengthening your uppermost arm away from your body.

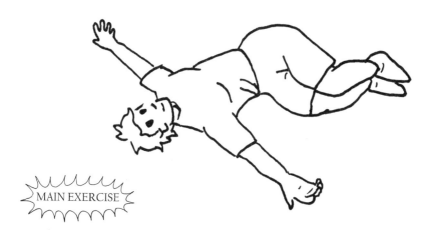

MAIN EXERCISE

CHAIR TWIST

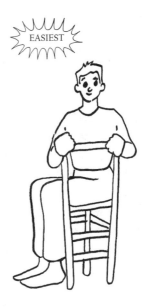

EASIEST

For this exercise you will need a chair with a firm bottom, a back, and no arms. A normal kitchen chair or firm office chair works fine. Sit sideways with the right side of your body against the back of the chair. Your feet are hip-width apart and pointing straight ahead. Your weight is evenly balanced on both sitting bones. Now turn your upper body so that the front of your body faces toward the back of the chair; grasp the back portion of the chair to help twist yourself. Your should feel the twist in your hips and your upper shoulders and back. Keep your body upright and your shoulders level. Don't let yourself sag. Focus on twisting your upper body.

Hold for thirty seconds to one minute. Repeat on the opposite side.

CROCODILE TWIST

Lie on your back with your legs straight and your arms at your side. Keeping your legs straight, place your right heel on top of your left toes so that your feet are stacked one on top of the other. While keeping your shoulders flat on the ground, twist your legs and your hips to the left bringing your stacked feet down toward the floor. *Keep your legs straight.* You should feel a deep stretch from your ankles up the sides of your legs and into your hips. Try turning your head gently to the opposite side (to the right).

Hold for thirty seconds, then repeat on the other side. The key to this exercise is to attempt to keep your legs straight and only twist as far as you can while maintaining good alignment.

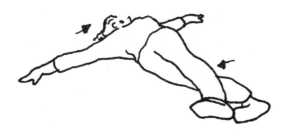

STANDING BENT-KNEE CHAIR TWIST

This is a little bit tricky to get set up properly, but it is one of my favorites because it allows you to calibrate the correct amount of stretch just for you.

Set a hard-bottomed chair at a forty-five degree angle and about three feet away from an outside corner of a room or doorway. Stand facing the chair and place your right foot up on the chair. Keep your hips square and your body lifted. Your left foot remains flat on the floor facing straight ahead. Next, turn to the right, reach behind you, and place your hand against the corner or hold onto the doorway.

This is where you may have to adjust the position of the chair—both the angle and distance—to make it just right for you. Your outstretched arm should be straight at shoulder level and you should feel the stretch in your right shoulder and hips. Without bending or tilting your hips, concentrate on turning your right shoulder outward. Gently push against your right outer knee with your left hand to rotate your hips in the opposite direction. Lift slightly upward.

Hold for one minute and repeat on the other side. The key to this stretch is to adjust the position and angle of the chair to maximize the stretch for you, to keep your hips facing straight ahead and to gently 'crank' the twist with your hand.

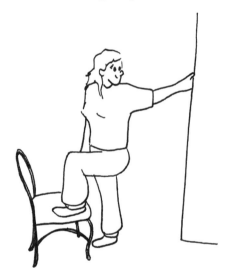

In the final chapter, you'll find out what else
you can do to maintain your alignment and
function in the years to come.

CHAPTER 8

What Else Can You Do

That which is used develops,
that which is not used wastes away.

– Hippocrates

Small changes in the way we think now can have enormous effects in our lives as they are played out over months and years. What may seem like an almost insignificant change in your thinking now, can make all the difference in the world in your health, years from now.

> When we change the way we think,
> we change our lives.

Many of our beliefs about health and fitness are based on the sketchiest of data—what a high school coach told us years ago, what we read in a popular bestseller during our formative years, or simply how we think things should be. Hopefully this book has challenged some of those beliefs. By now you should be aware of the downward spiral we are all prey to if we don't do something about it. You should have some idea about how muscles and bones work and the importance of postural alignment and keeping active in staying functional and preventing disability.

Here are some key new beliefs—new ways of thinking that can have a dramatic effect on your life now and in the years to come.

Eleven New Ways Of Thinking

1. *Become curious about posture. Place a high priority on postural alignment as one of your main fitness goals.*

That's what this book is about. Look around. Become aware of posture and alignment. Notice how people stand, sit, and move. Notice how young or old they are. Listen to their comments on what they can and cannot do. Listen to their physical complaints. Think about how much of this might have something to do with their alignment and lack of movement.

In your own fitness or health program, place a high priority on aligning yourself. Go for symmetry—one side equals the other. It is the imbalances in muscle strength and flexibility that cause problems down the road. The exercises in this book aren't the only exercises for postural alignment. They are a start; they are tools. Be open to finding new exercises, modifying existing exercises, and finding other resources that incorporate the same principles. Remember, postural alignment is the missing link to staying functional and preventing disability.

2. *Anything you do is going to help.*

This is the basic principle of this book. Anything you do to improve your postural alignment is going to help. Anything you do to keep active is going to help. There are truly no survivors on this earth. This book isn't about attaining some mythical perfect posture. Posture Alignment *will* improve your appearance. But it is also about maintaining function and preventing disability as long as possible.

If you only do one exercise for now, great. If you do more, fine. If all you do right now is change a few of your beliefs, that's okay too. Of course, I hope you'll eventually want to do more, but I know that by making one small change, or just starting to do *something* it can make a difference.

Remember, sometimes even a slight improvement in your alignment may be enough to take the pressure off of a joint or relieve muscle tension. A little improvement in alignment, a little more activity may prevent arthritis or the need for surgery now or five or ten years from now. Getting your shoulders back may be enough to make you look younger and more upright. Improving your alignment will make it more fun and less of a strain to be active.

3. *NOW is a good time to start.*

It doesn't matter how old you are, how fat you are, or how out of shape you are. It doesn't matter how crooked or straight your posture is. It doesn't matter whether you presently exercise or haven't exercised in a long time. It doesn't matter if your bones creak and your muscles ache. There is great power in beginnings, in taking that first step.

4. *Take every opportunity to move.*

This new belief requires a 180-degree shift in the way many of us think. We often think of movement as something to be avoided.

> Movement, any movement, has to
> be seen as something we need to do.

Regardless of your postural alignment, moving is always better than not moving. Our bodies crave movement and thrive when given enough of it. Remember, we live in a society that is becoming more and more motionless. When you can, walk instead of ride; take the stairs instead of the elevator. Do something the physical way instead of always relying on technology. Rage against the loss of motion in your life.

> The important thing isn't just to park your
> car farther away than you normally would
> and walk—it is knowing why in this day
> and age you have to do that.

At home, rather than paying for someone to do a simple job, or getting the most new-fangled gadget to do it, consider doing it yourself. Consider painting, raking, sweeping, scraping, lifting, hauling, pounding, shoveling. All of these activities provide much needed stimulus to often under-used muscles. They are as good for you as any exercise class. As you keep your house and yard up, you'll be keeping yourself up.

5. *Take every opportunity to move in varied ways.*

This is the corollary of the above principle. If movement is good, varied movement or moving in ways we don't usually move is better. Get out of the box. Take every opportunity to move in ways you don't usually move or aren't usually required to move: reach overhead, bend down, crawl, play with kids, climb, dance, stretch, bend over and under, do anything—different.

> ## If you don't usually move that way, then you should.

Here are some related suggestions:

• Activities that require movement in a variety of directions and angles are better than ones where you move in a simple repetitive manner.
• Do activities that use your whole body rather than just a few parts, e.g. play basketball or tennis rather than always jogging.
• Barring severe pollution, get outside. Sun, fresh air, and varied temperatures all have positive effects on your body.
• Given a choice, pick activities where you have to walk or move over varied terrain, for example, walk or bicycle outside up and down hills rather than on a stationary machine or someplace flat.

And it follows from this that . . .

6. *When given an opportunity to try a new sport, or do some physical activity you don't usually do, do it!*

When someone asks you to participate in a sport you don't usually do—golf, ping pong, tennis, badminton, swimming, dancing . . . bowling. Go! When you get the opportunity to fix or make something with your hands or use your whole body—do it. Whenever you can, take advantage of doing physical activities you don't usually get to do.

One measure for doing any activity should be:

> ## Will this activity provide my body with varied movement that it is not normally getting?

If the answer is yes, go for it. Rather than worrying about how good or bad you might perform, think of giving your body a dose of varied movement. Stimulate muscles and parts that may not usually get much stimulation and help prevent them from shutting down completely.

7. *Listen to your own body.*

We often become numb to our own bodies. In this age of experts, of talk-show hosts, of fitness experts (me?), of people who seemingly know more than we do, it is easy to become disconnected from our own bodies, from our own selves. It is easy not to trust ourselves or what we are feeling or what our bodies are telling us.

> ## Listen to your own body. Listen to your own self.

You know and you will always know your own body better than anyone else. And if you do the exercises, your awareness and kinesthetic sense will increase. Listen to it. You have an intuitive sense of correct alignment. You will feel what is tight and what has to be opened up. You will come to know which exercises are having the desired effect. You will know when you are ready to move on to more challenging exercises. And it follows from this . . .

8. *Be wary of allowing others to usurp your power and authority over yourself particularly when it comes to your musculoskeletal health.*

You have a very personal stake in your muscle and joint health and function. Become educated. Ask questions. Read. Don't always assume that the most complicated, technologically-advanced solutions are always the best. There are simple rules that govern the body's function. Learn them, use them.

> ## Don't play the game of helpless victim with regard to your muscle and joint health.

9. *Take a few opportunities throughout the day to consciously stand, sit, and move in an aligned manner.*

Waiting in line at the grocery store or for an elevator is a good opportunity to assume correct standing posture: feet hip-width apart pointing straight ahead, abdomen tucked in slightly, weight evenly distributed on both feet, chest lifted, head upright, shoulders lifted up, back, and then down (see Eight Images for Posture Alignment later in this chapter). Time spent in functional alignment is money in the bank or, if that doesn't appeal to you, money in a high-yielding investment that can't go down and is not affected by recession or other economic changes.

Do the same thing when you are sitting. Every hour or so for at least a minute, focus on sitting upright: weight evenly balanced on both hips, back lifted with a slight arch, shoulders back, head lifted, belly tucked. When walking up or down stairs, make it a point to try to walk with your feet pointing straight ahead.

As I've said before, doing these things alone won't cure all your postural ills. However, they will help remind your body of correct alignment and combined with the exercises, a battle will begin to be fought between your old way of standing, sitting, and moving and your new aligned way. Eventually the new way will win out.

10. *Don't let your age or your perceived competence in a sport keep you from participating.*

Recently I was at a tennis club and I happened to wander over to where four women were playing doubles. One was massively overweight. But when she was able to lumber over to where the ball was, she returned it with a wicked forehand. Her partner was in her sixties. Between them, they had almost every postural alignment defect in this book. All their curves and lines certainly weren't in the right places but they both played with a ferocious intensity.

Their opponents were similar—a tiny woman maybe five feet tall partnered with an elderly, overweight woman. These were not the people we see in the U.S. Open tennis championships. But they were playing with competitiveness appropriate to their ability. Each point was bitterly contested. And they were enjoying themselves and having fun. And moving!

It made me think of how many women (and men) of their size, shape, and age were at home right now ensconced in front of a television, or simply afraid to get out there and do something because they weren't good enough. "What would people think? I'm no good at this."

In this culture our obsession with winning and the access to seeing truly remarkable athletes in their sports has a tendency to turn off many a common man or woman from participating at all. After all, if you're not that good at it or can't be an expert, why bother?

But that is exactly the type of belief that puts and keeps you on the downward spiral. Who cares what anybody thinks of you? Who cares if you ever win a game or a point? Your goal in all this is to get out there and move. Because, if you don't, you are going to end up being the bigger loser.

Don't underestimate the value of competition. Sports, games, keeping score—they are all things that can help take our minds off the physical activity we are getting. Use this to your advantage.

11. *If you do have a favorite sport, watch your alignment.*

For those who spend hours doing a particular activity, make sure you aren't rein-forcing faulty alignment. Get correct instruction and always place correct funda-mentals and alignment before winning. In the long run, you will win more.

Also, if you have a favorite sport, make sure you are doing something to main-tain the parts of your body that may not be getting much of a workout from your chosen activity. The exercises in this book provide a perfect supplement.

Extending And Lengthening

In our society we often spend a great deal of time bending over a computer, a desk, or a steering wheel or engaged in other activities where we lean or hunch forward. With these activities our muscles tend to shorten and our shoulders, spines, and pelvises tend to round forward contributing to hunched and shorter stature partic-ularly as we get older. We close in on ourselves.

Thus, it becomes important in any exercise program and throughout our daily lives to emphasize activities that open our bodies up and lengthen them. Extension refers to opening up our joints such as straightening our arms, stretching our legs, knees, ankles, and feet straight to their full length, and opening up and stretching our back and shoulders backward.

Lengthening refers to consciously stretching our joints outward once they are extended. That is, don't just straighten your arm but stretch it as if you were trying to reach something just out of reach. Feel your arm pulling away from your shoulder, your forearm pulling away from your elbow, and your wrist and fingers stretch-ing out as long as possible.

Take every opportunity throughout the day to extend and lengthen as many times as you can.

Eight Images For Posture Alignment

Here are eight useful, fun images to help remind you of correct alignment. When we have a picture or image in our minds, our bodies readily conform to it. Use these images to supplement the Posture Alignment exercises. Use them while you're waiting in line, walking, or sitting at your desk.

Also sometimes we all just need a posture fix —a few second adjustment to our posture before an important meeting, an interview, or date. These can help.

1. *"Okay, Let's See How Tall You Are."* Remember when you were a kid and someone was measuring your height. Maybe you were at school or just competing with a friend standing back to back to see who was the tallest. Amazingly, this phrase produces a good approximation of perfect posture. We tend to lift ourselves up; pull our shoulders up and relax them back and lift our heads in a nice vertical line. Anytime you're standing around and slouching or want to look your best, just ask yourself, "Okay, let's see how tall you are."

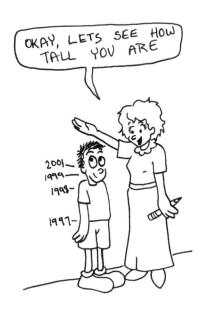

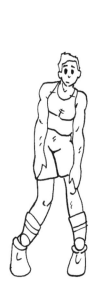

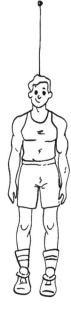

2. *String From The Top Of Your Head*
Imagine a string attached to the crown of your head extending you gently upward. The slight pull upward aligns your spine and hips. Your shoulders relax. This is another good image to use while waiting in line or for the elevator. What? You aren't taking the stairs!

3. *A Stack Of Blocks* Remember playing with blocks as children. In order for a stack of blocks not to fall, they all have to be lined up. Imagine the different segments of your body (head, chest, pelvis, legs) as blocks. Are they carelessly placed one on top of the other hopelessly leaning to one side or the other? Now, stack them up carefully, one on top of the other, beginning with your feet and ending with your head.

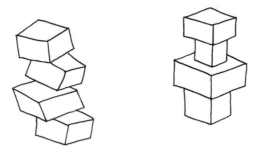

4. *Mountain Pose* This is the name for the basic standing pose in yoga. In this pose you simply stand. Your feet are together or hip-width apart, whatever is most comfortable for you, and pointing straight ahead. Your weight is evenly balanced on both feet side to side and front to back. Your waist and chest are *lifted*. Your shoulders are raised up, back, and then relaxed down. Your face is calm and relaxed. Think of yourself like a mountain—sturdy, strong, balanced, and grounded.

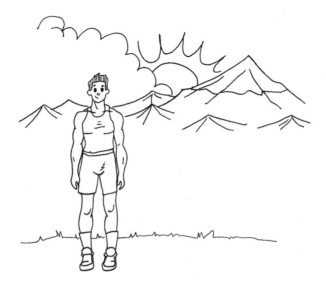

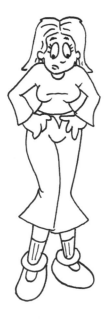

5. *Putting On A Tight Pair Of Jeans* Hopefully, once you get into shape they won't be tight for very long. Anyway, you know the feeling when you are trying to squeeze into a pair of tight jeans. You pull your abdomen in. This is a useful image to suggest the slight amount of tone you want in your lower abdomen with standing or sitting. Eventually this will become natural; meaning you won't have to think about it. It is a lifting-up feeling. The abdomen isn't tight, but "energized."

6. *Sitting On Your Throne* Imagine yourself as a king or queen sitting on your throne—upright, poised, confident, in control yet gently relaxed. That is the feeling you want when you are sitting. Focus on your weight being equally felt on both of your sitting bones. After all, if you slouch, none of your subjects will listen to you.

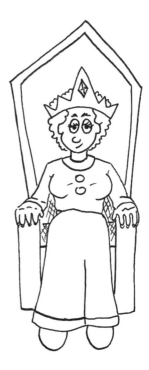

7. *Chariots Of Fire* Our body is like a chariot and our legs are like the two horses pulling the chariot. If one or both feet or legs are pointing to the sides, it makes it difficult for the chariot to go effectively forward. Both feet should point straight ahead or close to it. Otherwise, how can you expect to win the race at the coliseum?

Another variation on this is to think of your feet as the tires on a car. Both need to point straight ahead. If one or both point out to the side, it means you need alignment.

You can even imagine that song "Chariots of Fire" playing in the background as you walk.

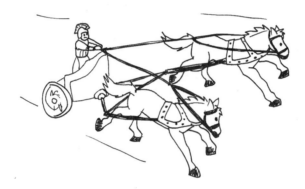

8. *Dots On Your Shoulders* Imagine a dot placed on the sides of each shoulder exactly equal distance from the front and back of your body. Ideally, a shirt seam should run directly across the top of your shoulders, and the dots would be placed where the seam meets the sides of your shoulders. Are your shoulders rolled forward so that the dots are pointing more forward than out to the sides? Use this image to help remind you to pull your shoulders back so that the dots point more to the sides.

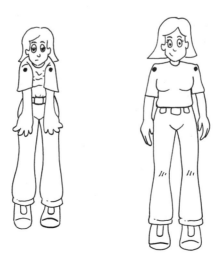

Other things you can do . . .

Take A Yoga Class

Yoga is one of the best overall exercise activities readily available in most communities. Yoga has had a resurgence in great part due to its soft, gentle nature and the recognition of the need for balancing strength and flexibility as we grow older. The yoga postures complement the exercises of Posture Alignment; in fact, many of the Posture Alignment exercises are taken directly from yoga.

The difference between Posture Alignment and yoga is that Posture Alignment makes it its goal to identify and correct alterations in alignment, while yoga uses more of a shotgun approach. Often the specific exercises ordinary people need most aren't done enough in the average yoga class to correct their problems.

That said, I heartily recommend yoga in all its forms. And if you already practice yoga and add the Posture Alignment exercises, your yoga practice will improve dramatically. The following are some of the advantages of yoga:

• *Yoga is a gradual process.* The poses build on each other. You start off with simple postures and develop the necessary muscular strength and flexibility before moving on to more advanced poses.

• *Yoga addresses both sides of the body.* Whatever is done on one side is done on the other. This encourages balance and symmetry. Discrepancies in strength or flexibility become readily apparent.

• *Yoga's variety of postures addresses all major muscle groups and joints.*

• *Yoga is fun.*

• *Yoga is devoid of competition.* We often have enough unnecessary competition in our lives. Yoga offers a respite from this.

• *Yoga is generally practiced in a quiet, almost introspective atmosphere.* It allows one to become more aware of one's body. It rekindles our kinesthetic sense.

• *Yoga is personal.* Yoga honors individual differences and promotes listening to oneself and one's own body.

Weight Lifting

Using weights to become stronger is like using industrial strength chemicals. They are powerful; you have to be careful and know what you are doing.

That said, we are all generally much weaker than we think. Our muscle weakness sneaks up on us. Once you are in good alignment or close to it, weights can help strengthen the muscles that keep you in correct alignment.

Make sure you get some instruction if you are new to using weights, and make sure you are meticulous in your technique. The time to stop lifting or doing a given exercise is when you start to compensate, that is, when you start bending and weaving and using muscles not assigned to the task.

Whether using hand-held weights or using weight machines at a health club, using enough weight to do 10-15 repetitions is adequate. Doing a supplemental weight-lifting program two or three times a week is enough, since you need to give your body an opportunity to recover between workouts.

The drawback to weight training by itself is that it doesn't always address all the little muscles that we need and use. And really what we are after is function, not just making our biceps or quads strong.

If you already participate in a weight-lifting program and are significantly out of alignment, you may consider putting your weight-lifting program on hold for awhile. Or take a close look at your regimen and emphasize those exercises that complement your postural alignment goal. For example, if your shoulders are rolled forward, it makes more sense to do exercises which open up the front of the chest and strengthen the muscles in the back and between the shoulder blades, than to do those that tighten and constrict the muscles in the front of the chest.

We all naturally lose muscle mass and bone density to varying degrees as we age. Post-menopausal women in particular are prone to osteoporosis (bone-thinning leading to an increased incidence of fractures) and weight lifting has been shown to obviate some of the risk for this.

Sports and Other Physical Activities

I am an advocate of any and all sports and physical activities. The only caveat is this: if your alignment is way off, you may not improve your alignment as quickly as you'd like if you continue doing a sport or activity that demands that you move in a non-aligned way or use your old compensations.

See, on one hand, you may be doing the Posture Alignment exercises, which move your body in a whole new direction, and then you go back and run umpteen miles and your style of running reinforces your old way of moving. As talked about in Chapter 3, our bodies add up all the stimuli given them and that determines our alignment. You could be like a man or woman caught between two worlds.

So, be wary. If you are significantly out of alignment, it might be reasonable to cut back a little on your primary sport until you move closer to correct alignment.

Once you are in good alignment, virtually any sport, exercise class, or activity is okay.

Rolfing

Rolfing is a form of body work in which the practitioner performs a form of deep tissue massage allegedly breaking up connective tissue and allowing the body to reconstitute itself in a more integrated and aligned manner.

Posture Alignment shares much of the philosophy and many of the underlying principles of Rolfing. Although expensive (ten sessions are recommended and cost around $100 each), for those with the money I believe it is useful adjunct to Posture Alignment.

The Grace Period

Life often provides us with a grace period when it comes to our health. We can go for years and years and not have any problems. Our bodies often work in the background like faithful servants not demanding any attention. We often don't appreciate or notice our muscle and joint health until something goes amiss.

But after a certain age, this changes. We begin to experience changes in our physical functioning. We see and hear about problems in others our age. We watch as others begin to slide to varying degrees down the slippery slope of the downward spiral.

At this stage, there is a fork in the road. We reach a point—again, often because of the nature of our jobs and society—where we have to do something to maintain our physical health or risk sliding down that slope ourselves. At this point people generally divide themselves into two categories: those that are doing something about it and those who aren't. You now know the importance of postural alignment and have some tools—exercises and new ways of thinking—to help maintain your posture and function. After reading this book, I am sure you will be one of the people who will be doing something about it.

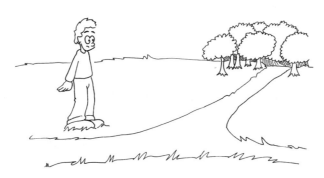

> After a certain age, you are either doing something to maintain your movement function or you are not. It's that simple.

Final Exam:

Your friend asks you to go play tennis with them. You don't play tennis. You should . . .

    a. make up an excuse why you can't go.

    b. highly consider going with them because of the varied movement it will provide your body.

    c. tell them it's not your sport and to get someone else.

Something falls on the floor under the table. You should . . .

    a. leave it there. Let someone else pick it up.

    b. disregard it completely.

    c. use your best Reaching Down Under Lunge (Page 164) and pick it up.

Your knee hurts. You think you have arthritis. You see your doctor and listen to his or her advice. Along with that, you should also. . .

    a. push for surgery as soon as possible. After all, everyone in your family has weak knees.

    b. highly consider the possibility that once the acute event is over, you may need to strengthen the muscles in your lower extremities, and work on your alignment.

You don't have time to do any of the silly exercises in this book. You should . . .

    a. buy another book that fits better with what you are willing or able to do.

    b. not do anything. After all, if you can't do everything in the book, why bother.

    c. stay active as much as possible in order to maintain function and prevent muscle and joint problems. Consider doing one or two of the exercises when you do have the time.

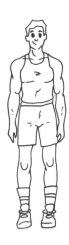
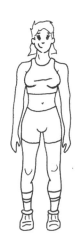

ORDER
POSTURE ALIGNMENT
NOW

Please send me _____ copies of *Posture Alignment - The Missing Link in Health and Fitness* at $19.95 each plus $3.50 shipping and handling for the first book and $.50 for each additional book (Colorado residents add 2.9% sales tax; El Paso County residents add additional 1% sales tax, and City of Colorado Springs residents yet an additional 2.5% sales tax). Please allow 15 days for delivery (usually much shorter).

My check or money order for $ _____ is enclosed.

Name _____

Address _____

City/State/ Zip _____

Phone _____

Please make check payable to and return this form to:

Marcellina Mountain Press
P. O. Box 6781
Colorado Springs, CO 80934

For credit card orders call: 1-800-431-1579

Or visit our website: www.posturealignment.com

Retailers or distributors, please contact us for discounts.